DRUG TRUTHS

DRUG TRUTHS
DISPELLING THE MYTHS ABOUT PHARMA R&D

JOHN L. LAMATTINA, Ph.D.

OCT 07 2009

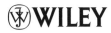

WILEY

A JOHN WILEY & SONS, INC., PUBLICATION

Published by John Wiley & Sons, Inc., Hoboken, New Jersey
Published simultaneously in Canada

For general information on our other products and services or for technical support, please contact our Customer Care Department within the United States at (800) 762-2974, outside the United States at (317) 572-3993 or fax (317) 572-4002.

Wiley also publishes its books in a variety of electronic formats. Some content that appears in print may not be available in electronic formats. For more information about Wiley products, visit our web site at www.wiley.com.

Library of Congress Cataloging-in-Publication Data:

LaMattina, John L.
   Drug truths : dispelling the myths about pharma R&D / John L. LaMattina.
      p. ; cm.
   Includes bibliographical references and index.
   ISBN 978-0-470-39318-5 (cloth)
      1. Drug development–United States.   2. Pharmaceutical industry–United States.   3. Drugs–Research–United States.   I. Title.
      [DNLM: 1. Drug Industry–economics–United States.   2. Drug Design–United States.
   3. Research Design–United States. QV 736 L217d 2009]
      RM301.25L36 2009
      615′.19—dc22

                                                                                    2008033272

Printed in the United States of America

10 9 8 7 6 5 4 3

For Mary

CONTENTS

ACKNOWLEDGMENTS

THIS BOOK is based on the efforts and dedication of thousands of scientists from around the globe who use their talents every day to invent new medicines to treat the scourges of the world. We owe all of these people our respect and admiration. They are the ones on whom we depend to help cure us.

I am particularly indebted to the many Pfizer scientists who worked on the many projects described herein that helped to push back medical and scientific boundaries. I am especially grateful to colleagues who provided their insights and comments, including: for Lipitor, David Canter and Roger Newton; for torcetrapib, Steve Ryder, Chuck Shear, Mark Bamberger and Roger Ruggeri; for CP-690,550, Paul Changelian and Ethan Weiner; for Chantix, Jim Heym, Marty Jefson, Dave Schulz, and Jotham Coe; for Selzentry, Pat Dorr, Chris Hitchcock, Mike Westby, Howie Mayer, and Mike Dunne; for Zoloft, Gary Ryan; for Celebrex, Karen Seibert and Ken Verburg; for Viagra, Mike Allen and Ian Osterloh; and for the Pfizer Oncology programs, Mike Morin and Chuck Baum.

In addition, I am grateful to John Swen, Joe Hammang, Sue Anderson, Lydia Pan, and Eric Utt for their insights on the criticisms routinely levied against Big Pharma.

Finally, three people were incredibly helpful in the preparation of this book: Stephen Lederer and Justin McCarthy, for their insightful editorial comments; and Donna Green, who miraculously pulled this all together.

INTRODUCTION

FOR MANY scientists a job in the Research and Development labs of a pharmaceutical company is a dream come true. After having gone to school for many years (more than 20 for some with Ph.D.s), scientists are finally able to utilize their talent and training in an organization where they can immediately act on their ambition to make a difference in the discovery and development of new medicines.

I knew from an early age that I wanted to be a chemist. I found the science involved in building complex molecules fascinating. Like the "baby boomers" of the late 1960s, I wanted to "make a difference." Working on the creation of molecules that potentially had important biological activity was very appealing. I pictured myself working in state-of-the-art laboratory facilities and having access to the finest equipment and technology available. I envisioned working with outstanding scientists from around the globe, all of whom would bring their special talents to bear on projects designed to produce new drugs to treat the scourges of mankind: cancer, Alzheimer's disease, heart disease, life-threatening bacterial and fungal infections, and so on.

I majored in chemistry at Boston College, where I received a B.S. degree in 1971. From there I entered the Ph.D. program at the University of New Hampshire, where I studied organic chemistry with Professor Robert E. Lyle. At UNH I specialized in the chemistry of heterocyclic molecules—the type of molecules that make up the vast majority of medicines. After graduating from UNH in 1975, I went on to Princeton University as a National Institutes of Health post-doctoral fellow, where I studied with Professor Edward C. Taylor, one of the leading heterocyclic organic chemists in the world. By 1977 I was ready for a job in the "real world" and I was fortunate enough to join Pfizer's Research and Development laboratory in Groton, Connecticut. Despite the many years of schooling that I had, I quickly found that I knew little when it came to the discovery of new drugs. I was fortunate, however, to be surrounded by experts in not just chemistry but also biology, toxicology, drug metabolism, and other key disciplines. While these early days were challenging, they were intellectually invigorating. I was working with great scientists committed to curing the world's diseases.

Interestingly, scientists aren't the only ones who relish the experience of working in such an environment. Being a part of this enterprise is sought by many others who play key roles, such as computer experts who design the systems needed to track and analyze data and facilities professionals who help in designing and maintaining laboratories that maximize efficiencies. Hundreds and hundreds of people are involved in this discovery and development process and, when a new medicine is approved by the regulatory agencies around the globe, all take tremendous pride in their respective contributions.

Not too long ago a cancer patient visited the Pfizer Groton labs to thank the people there for literally saving his life. He was diagnosed with malignant melanoma in 2002. The two most promising treatment options that existed then had both failed. His cancer was spreading and doctors gave him two months to live. In 2004 he entered an experimental study with a new Pfizer drug. His results are best described in his own words:

"I could have been dead in April of 2004 without this drug," he told an audience more than two years later. "Each day I have had since has been an extraordinary gift. I wanted to come here to say thank you to each and every person. I don't care if you're working on anti-CTLA4 or not. With these tools you can't tell which of them is going to turn into something so important for someone in your family or a neighbor. So now I feel it's my job to remind you folks of how important what you're doing really is. And it is a tough time to be working in the pharmaceutical development industry. I know what's going on, I know the heat that you get. Let it go, and just focus on the benefit that you are providing. You should be able to go home and sleep at night, thinking, you know, this was a pretty good day."

This patient's words were both inspirational and motivating. To help people like him is what brings these scientists to work every day.

One would hope that this patient's view of the work done in pharmaceutical R&D would be shared by many others and valued highly. Unfortunately, that is not the case. Headlines about this industry during the last 10 years have questioned what contributions are really made by these scientists. It is not unusual to read stories claiming that drugs are not discovered by "Big Pharma" but rather that the true discoveries are made in academic or government labs or that the industry wastes resources by focusing on "me too" drugs. The innovation of these same scientists is often challenged with claims that real innovation occurs only in the biotech sector of the industry. Pharmaceutical R&D is even accused of inventing diseases in order to turn a profit. *None of these claims are true.*

Furthermore, such uninformed views are not just aggravating but are also insulting to the thousands of people in the pharmaceutical industry who dedicate their professional lives to discovering new medicines. The R&D carried out in pharmaceutical companies is critical in the overall advancement of medical science. In fact, one might argue that it provides the crucial link because it is the work of pharmaceutical R&D that actually proves or disproves medical hypotheses that result in new treatments or cures.

If this is true, why isn't the important role of this research universally recognized? There are many reasons for the current state of affairs, but the primary reason is a lack of understanding of what pharmaceutical R&D actually does, how technically difficult it is, what the process entails, and how long and costly the drug discovery and development process really is. Not too long ago, I was able to see this problem first hand.

In March 2006, I was asked to be the Harold A. Iddles lecturer of the Chemistry Department at the University of New Hampshire. This was a great thrill for me and I accepted this opportunity excitedly. For one thing, I myself had listened to Iddles lecturers some 30 years earlier as a graduate student at UNH, hearing some of the outstanding chemists in the world such as Nobel Laureate Robert Merrifield. To be asked to now actually be an Iddles lecturer myself was an honor I had never envisioned.

But there was another intriguing aspect to this opportunity. One of the requirements for an Iddles lecturer was for one of the lectures to be a presentation of a general nature, one that would be of interest not just to the UNH community but also to people in the southeast New Hampshire region as well. The title of this talk was "Pharmaceutical R&D: The Worlds' Hope for Tomorrow's Cures." Some of the questions addressed in this talk included:

- What value do new medicines bring to society?
- Where do medicines come from?
- What innovation does Big Pharma bring?
- How are risks and benefits of medicines evaluated?

This 45-minute talk began at 4 PM to an audience of a few hundred people. The question and answer period that followed lasted another hour and a quarter when the meeting organizers had to end it. Nothing like this had ever been seen before at an Iddles lecture. The questions covered the entire spectrum of what is done in Pharmaceutical R&D. People were more than curious—they had dozens of questions and wanted answers. They were stunned to hear how long and costly it is to discover new drugs. People had little appreciation of the cutting edge science involved in pharmaceutical R&D. They asked how scientists stay motivated when, after spending years on a program, it suddenly dies. By 6 PM, it became pretty clear that the audience suddenly had another view of what pharmaceutical companies did, the challenges they face, and, most importantly, the critical nature of their work in bringing forward new medicines. The audience began to see a major piece of the health care debate in a totally new light.

This curiosity is not unique to this group of people in New Hampshire. Everyone expects something from the drug industry. If the industry doesn't deliver, people take it personally. Is there any other industry in which this is true?

Physicians and patients, investors, regulators, and administrators all have an active interest in the drug industry. Everyone wants to know what makes drugs work medically and economically. Why are drugs so expensive? Why do drugs take so long to develop? Is it the drug companies or investors who demand high profits? Does patient safety really take a back seat to profits?

This book attempts to answer these questions by focusing on the discovery and development of important new medicines. In effect, it paints an insider's account of the pharmaceutical industry drug discovery process, the very real costs of misperceptions about the industry, the high stakes—both economic and scientific—of developing drugs, the triumphs that come when new compounds reach the market and save lives, and the despair that follows when new compounds fail. It is hoped that this book will broaden the views of many readers as happened with the UNH audience.

Why is this important? To the extent that the misperceptions of pharmaceutical R&D continue, overall healthcare is undermined. As the reader will see in the ensuing chapters, major new treatments for AIDS, heart disease, nicotine addition, rheumatoid arthritis, and others have emerged solely from this industry. Eroding of support for pharmaceutical R&D will result in delays for the discovery and development of even better new medicines. Ironically, this is coming at a time when medical science has unprecedented opportunities thanks to the unraveling of the human genome.

Finally, the Presidential election in 2008 will again thrust the pharmaceutical industry into the spotlight. The value of medicines and the importance of pharmaceutical R&D will be debated and will undoubtedly be scrutinized as a new President takes over in 2009. It is now a critical time to level the playing field.

PART *I*

A MATTER
OF THE HEART

IN THE 1990s, work from a number of academic laboratories suggested that infection with a certain pathogen, *Chlamydia pneumoniae*, might play a role in the development of coronary artery disease. The scientific evidence for this was intriguing. For one thing, blood analysis of patients with heart disease showed evidence of prior *C. pneumoniae* infection. In addition, multiple studies showed that this organism was actually present in atherosclerotic plaques. Finally, animal studies showed that infection with *C. pneumoniae* accelerated the development of atherosclerosis.

That a pathogen like *C. pneumoniae* could play a role in heart disease wasn't far-fetched. The atherosclerotic process is initiated by inflammatory processes and bacteria are known to be a cause of such events. Furthermore, the role of bacteria in noninfectious diseases has precedence. Dr. Barry Marshall won the Nobel Prize for his work in showing that such a pathogen, *Helicobacter pylori*, was the cause of peptic and gastric ulcers, thereby leading to new methods of treating gastrointestinal disease.

Early clinical trials of preventative antibiotic treatment in patients with heart disease provided mixed results. These studies were deemed to be of too short duration or too small in terms of numbers of patients to see an effect on reducing heart attacks. Thus, in the late 1990s, three large-scale long-term studies were begun to get an answer to the relevance of *C. pneumoniae* in cardiovascular disease.

The first study was the "Weekly Intervention with Zithromax for Atherosclerosis and Its Related Disorders" (WIZARD).[1] In WIZARD, 7747 patients who had suffered a previous myocardial infarction were randomized to receive either azithromycin (Zithromax) on a weekly basis for 12 weeks or a placebo. These patients were then monitored for a year while looking for a reduction in cardiovascular events such as recurrent fatal or nonfatal heart attacks, hospitalization for bypass surgery, balloon angioplasty, or angina. The result: at the end of 12 months, there was no difference in cardiac outcomes between patients who took azithromycin as compared to placebo.

Perhaps to see the desired effect, azithromycin needed to be dosed for a longer period of time and patients needed to be followed for more than one year to see the potential overall benefit. This was the basis for the ACES trial,[2] "The Azithromycin

Drug Truths: Dispelling the Myths About Pharma R&D, by John L. LaMattina
Copyright © 2009 John Wiley & Sons, Inc.

and Coronary Events Study." This trial, which involved 4012 patients, had a design that paralleled the WIZARD study except that patients were dosed for a year and then followed for 3.5 years. Unfortunately, the result for ACES was the same as in WIZARD: There was no significant risk reduction in heart attacks or strokes between azithromycin and placebo.

Finally the third study,[3] "Antibiotic treatment of *Chlamydia pneumoniae* after Acute Coronary Syndrome," was also conducted at this time using a different antibiotic, gatifloxacin. This trial enrolled 4162 patients who had recently been hospitalized with acute coronary syndrome. Patients were randomized to drug and placebo, but in this study the patients were given a monthly regimen of gatifloxacin for two years. After 30 months of follow-up at the end of the 2-year dosing period, again there was no difference between the antibiotic and placebo groups in terms of reducing cardiovascular events.

Why did these efforts to eradicate *C. pneumoniae* fail to provide a beneficial effect on heart disease? There is no clear answer. It is possible that the bacteria must be eradicated at the early stage of the process of atherogenesis before the disease fully sets in. However, these studies proved conclusively that antibiotics should not be recommended for treating coronary heart disease.

These studies involved hundreds of scientists and physicians from around the world and cost tens of millions of dollars, and they could only be accomplished with the novel antibiotics discovered by the pharmaceutical industry along with their resources of talent and funds. These clinical trials were designed jointly by industry scientists and clinicians along with their academic collaborators who performed these experiments at academic medical centers. However, the risk involved in terms of financing these studies rested solely in the lap of the pharmaceutical company sponsors. The *C. pneumoniae* story is a great example of the core contribution that the pharmaceutical industry makes to medicine: it proves or disproves medical hypotheses—in this case, that eradication of *C. pneumoniae* has no impact in preventing cardiovascular events.

Part one of this book focuses on these contributions with respect to cholesterol and heart disease. As you will see, when a medical hypothesis is proven, patients and pharmaceutical companies benefit. Likewise, when a medical hypothesis turns out to be incorrect, the disappointment can reverberate not just through companies but also through patients, physicians, and scientists.

CHAPTER 1

CHOLESTEROL DRUGS ARE UNNECESSARY

I**T IS** virtually impossible to go a day without being reminded of the relationship of heart disease and high cholesterol levels. While walking through grocery store aisles, you are hit with a variety of no-cholesterol, low-fat foods. Simply reading a magazine or watching television will expose you to advertisements warning of the dangers of high cholesterol resulting from diet or from poor genes. Drugs to treat high cholesterol, commonly known as statins, are the most highly prescribed drugs in history. Even the spokespeople for statin drugs, such as the inventor of the artificial heart, Dr. Robert Jarvik, have become highly scrutinized.

And yet, a little over 20 years ago, the relationship between heart disease and high cholesterol levels was unproven and largely ignored.[1] In fact, in 1989 *The Atlantic Monthly* featured an article entitled "The Cholesterol Myth," which said: "Lowering your cholesterol is next to impossible with diet, and often dangerous with drugs—and it will not make you live any longer."[2] Furthermore, if you had a total cholesterol level of 300 mg/deciliter (dL), you were considered to be on the upper end of normal. And no one had a clue as to their own relative ratios of high-density lipoproteins (HDL), the so-called "good" cholesterol, and low-density lipoproteins (LDL), the "bad" cholesterol. This began to change in the 1980s with the publication of a number of studies that began to provide concrete evidence that there was truly a causative role for cholesterol and particularly LDL cholesterol in heart attacks and strokes. One such study was the Framingham Heart Study.

This landmark study has been ongoing since 1948. It has been administered by the National Heart, Lung and Blood Institute of the NIH and was begun with over 5000 adults from Framingham, Massachusetts. Studying this population for 25 years enabled the identification of a number of risk factors for identifying potential victims of heart disease. These factors included smoking, excess weight, lack of exercise, stress, hypertension, and a high total cholesterol/HDL ratio.[3] While some of these risk factors were already well-accepted, the Framingham Study provided strong evidence that abnormal lipids were also a major risk factor.

At the same time, the results of another major study appeared. The Lipid Research Clinics Coronary Primary Prevention Trial (LRC-CPPT) studied the effects of lowering cholesterol levels in reducing heart disease in 3800 middle-aged asymptomatic men with high cholesterol.[4] These men were studied for seven years with half of the group on placebo and the other half on a compound called cholestyramine, a resin that acts as a bile acid sequestrant and thereby was known to lower cholesterol levels modestly. Both groups were on a moderate cholesterol-lowering diet. The results of this study proved convincing. The cholestyramine patients had their overall cholesterol lowered by 13% and their LDL cholesterol lowered by 20%, as compared to 5% and 8% for those on placebo. This lowering of cholesterol resulted in a 24% reduction in definite death due to heart disease, as well as reductions in heart attacks, angina, and coronary bypass surgeries. For the first time, proof was in hand that lowering total cholesterol and LDL cholesterol had a direct impact in reducing heart disease. These results were compelling enough that the NIH began to encourage physicians to teach patients about the importance of treating high cholesterol.[5]

While these data were encouraging, a major difficulty needed to be overcome. Cholestyramine was not a patient friendly medicine. Up to 20 grams of this drug needed to be taken in divided doses two to three times per day. These large doses tended to cause adverse gastrointestinal effects such as constipation, gas, and bloating. But the biggest hurdle for patients was taking the dose of medicine itself as it is an insoluble resin. It has been described as drinking liquid cement. Clearly, better-tolerated cholesterol-lowering medicines were needed.

At about this same time, a discovery was made that eventually revolutionized the treatment of heart disease. A Japanese microbiologist, Akira Endo at the Sankyo company in Tokyo, was searching fermentation broths of *Penicillium citrinum* for novel antimicrobial agents.[6] During this work he found a compound now known as compactin. This agent proved to be an inhibitor of an enzyme called HMG-CoA reductase. This enzyme is involved in the critical step in the body's synthesis of cholesterol. Ironically, compactin did not have useful antimicrobial activity. However, the potential for using this agent in controlling high cholesterol levels was recognized by Endo. Theoretically, if one could safely block the actions of HMG-CoA reductase, the biosynthesis of cholesterol would be reduced, thereby lowering total cholesterol.

Sankyo designed and managed a clinical trial to explore the effects of compactin in humans. This study showed that it did, in fact, effectively lower both total cholesterol and LDL cholesterol in patients who were genetically disposed to high plasma lipids.[7] Unfortunately, Sankyo had to suspend clinical trials with compactin due to unspecified adverse findings in animal studies.

Merck scientists were also actively pursuing this field of research, and their chemists discovered the HMG-CoA reductase inhibitor, lovastatin.[7] Lovastatin was shown to be safe in healthy volunteers and proved to be very effective in lowering total cholesterol and LDL cholesterol in patients with heart disease. The efficacy of lovastatin was elucidated by the Nobel Prize-winning work of Michael S. Brown and Joseph L. Goldstein, who showed that statins, by virtue of blockading cholesterol biosynthesis, improve the ability of the liver to remove LDL from the blood, thus making it less likely for LDL to deliver cholesterol to the artery wall.[8]

Lovastatin was launched by Merck under the trade name of Mevacor in 1987. They then followed this breakthrough with a superior statin, Zocor (generic name:

simvastatin) in 1991. Despite the availability of these two compounds, statins were still not universally prescribed in the early 1990s. The reason for this was twofold: First, physicians were reluctant to prescribe a drug that patients were to take for the rest of their lives without some assurances that long-term use of such drugs were indeed safe; second, while lowering cholesterol had beneficial effects in reducing the risk of heart disease, there was no evidence that long-term survival was enhanced. This all changed in 1994 with the publication of the results of the landmark Scandinavian Simvastatin Survival Study (4S).[9] In this study, 4444 patients who had a previous myocardial infarction and serum cholesterol of 215–310 mg/dL on a lipid-lowering diet were treated with either simvastatin or placebo for 5 years. Over this time period, simvastatin produced mean decreases of 25% in total cholesterol and 35% of LDL cholesterol. But more importantly, only 182 patients on simvastatin (out of 2221) had died as compared to 256 (out of 2223) on placebo—a statistically significant risk reduction of 30%. The controversy was over as was evidenced in an editorial in the *British Medical Journal* entitled "Lower Patients' Cholesterol Now."[10] Based on the 4S study and other examples, the authors concluded the following for patients with angina or with a previous myocardial infarction: "There is no longer any controversy about what to do for these patients and no justification for inertia."

Thus, by the mid-1990s the principle of lowering LDL cholesterol was established. Statins were by far the agents of choice to control high cholesterol. The safety and ease of administration of statins was such that these compounds became the biggest selling drugs of all time. But suddenly all of this was again challenged in 2008 with the announcement of the results of a clinical study known as ENHANCE.

ZETIA®: AN INHIBITOR OF DIETARY CHOLESTEROL ABSORPTION

Statins clearly are efficacious in lowering plasma cholesterol. However, one's cholesterol level is impacted not only by the body's synthesis of cholesterol but also by the amount of cholesterol and fat taken in through one's daily diet. Theoretically, a compound that could block the absorption of cholesterol in the digestive tract would lower plasma cholesterol.

Given that statins are so effective, why would one care about lowering cholesterol absorption in the gut? First of all, despite the tens of millions of people who are successfully treated with statins, not everyone can tolerate these drugs. A small minority of patients do experience side effects that prevent statin usage. This is not unusual. As will be discussed in subsequent chapters, *no* medication can be successfully used universally, not even aspirin. Thus, having an alternative to statins is important to those with high LDL cholesterol who cannot tolerate them. Second, in theory a cholesterol absorption inhibitor should be able to be used in combination with a statin because their mechanisms would be anticipated to be complementary. For those people with established heart disease and very high LDL cholesterol, the combination of a statin with a cholesterol absorption inhibitor could theoretically provide better control than a statin alone.

Scientists at Schering-Plough were successful in discovering and developing such a compound, namely, Zetia[11] (genetic name: ezetimibe). While not as potent as statins, Zetia lowers LDL cholesterol by 18% as a stand-alone agent. It was on the basis of this activity that the FDA approved Zetia.

It is important to note that, unlike the situation with cholestyramine, niacin, or statins, studies have not yet been published on the reduction of heart attacks or strokes with Zetia. The FDA approved Zetia on the basis of its ability to lower LDL cholesterol by more than 15%. Essentially, the FDA approved this drug on its effect on a surrogate marker. The FDA will give approval of new drugs on the basis of the drug's beneficial effect on well-established markers of disease. In the case of heart disease, given that the lowering of LDL cholesterol by three distinct mechanisms was shown to have great benefits for this sick population, the FDA established that novel lipid-lowering agents with unique mechanisms can also be approved provided that these agents lower LDL cholesterol by at least 15%. The FDA also requires that the manufacturer of such an agent conduct long-term studies post-approval to show the impact of this new compound on long-term outcomes such as heart attacks and strokes. However, given the strong scientific precedence in an area like this, it is felt that patients should have access to a compound that lowers LDL cholesterol in advance of the long-term outcome study results. Zetia certainly fit this paradigm.

The use of surrogate markers is not unique to the lipid-lowering field. For decades, high blood pressure has been used as a surrogate marker for heart disease and drugs have been approved solely for their ability to lower blood pressure in hypertensive patients. In the early treatment of AIDS, the FDA approved drugs on the basis of reducing the levels of human immunodeficiency virus (HIV), the virus that causes this disease. Improvements in bone mineral density scans are used as surrogates for osteoporosis. While long-term outcome studies are eventually required as ultimate proof of a drug's benefit, these can take 5–7 years to complete. Thus, surrogate markers, which are recognized and accepted by the medical community, are of value in bringing important new medicines to patients in a timely fashion.

VYTORIN® AND THE ENHANCE TRIAL

Although Zetia was an important medicine in its own right, Schering-Plough recognized that this agent would be combined with various statins. As part of their New Drug Application (NDA) filing, Schering-Plough included studies that combined Zetia with leading statins such as atorvastatin (Lipitor) and simvastatin (Zocor) to show that co-administration of Zetia was safe and that the LDL lowering of the combination was improved over the statin alone. Based on these data, it was obvious that there would be value in having a single pill that combined both types of agents. In recognition of this, Schering-Plough and Merck set up a joint venture to commercialize a new medicine that would combine this cholesterol absorption inhibitor with simvastatin. This new combination drug was called Vytorin,[12] and it was approved by the FDA in 2004.

The introduction of Vytorin was greeted with mixed reviews. Some physicians felt that the combination was a good idea. After all, evidence to date had supported the view that the lower one's LDL cholesterol was, the less likely the risk of cardiovascular disease would be. However, some cardiologists felt that there was no scientific evidence yet available to show that clinical events would be reduced using this combination as compared to using a statin alone. Until such information was in hand, these physicians felt that there was little need for Vytorin.

Schering-Plough and Merck recognized that full acceptance of Vytorin would not be realized unless such long-term cardiovascular outcome studies were successfully completed. And so, after the approval of Vytorin, a variety of studies were launched. One such study, IMPROVE-IT (IMProved Reduction of Outcomes: Vytorin Efficacy International Trial),[13] is a 5-year study involving 12,500 patients scheduled to be completed in 2011. It is designed to measure the effectiveness of Vytorin compared with simvastatin alone in reducing deaths due to any cardiovascular event.

Given that it will be years before the results of this study will be available, the joint venture has conducted other studies to attempt to show the value of the combination. One of these studies is the "Effect of Ezetimibe plus Simvastatin versus Simvastatin Alone on Atherosclerosis in the Carotid Artery" trial, commonly referred to as ENHANCE. The ENHANCE trial involved 720 patients with a relatively rare disease called heterozygous familial hypercholesterolemia (HeFH). Patients with HeFH have a reduced ability to remove LDL cholesterol from their circulation. As a result, they have LDL levels in excess of 400 mg/dL and are at high risk of atherosclerosis.

Approximately one person in 500 has HeFH. ENHANCE was an "imaging trial"—that is, a trial that didn't measure reduction of cardiovascular events but a trial that measured the thickness of the carotid arteries using vascular ultrasound. Theoretically, one would hope that the following scenario would occur:

1. The combination of a cholesterol absorption inhibitor with a statin (i.e., Vytorin) would provide greater LDL lowering than a statin alone.

2. This enhanced LDL lowering would result in less atherosclerosis in HeFH patients.

3. Less atherosclerosis would be a predictor of fewer heart attacks and strokes over an extended period of time.

That was the hope for ENHANCE. Unfortunately, science isn't always this straightforward. Analysis of the 30,000 ultrasound carotid artery images taken from these 720 patients proved more difficult than originally envisioned by the investigators, thereby delaying the final report of the ENHANCE results. This resulted in a great deal of speculation about the study and its outcome. As a result, Merck/Schering-Plough took the unusual step of issuing a press release[14] in advance of publishing the data. The press release indicated that there was no difference in the carotid arteries of patients on Vytorin versus those on simvastatin alone, despite the fact that after 2 years the Vytorin group had LDL cholesterol reductions of 58% as compared to 41% for simvastatin. The full results of the ENHANCE trial have subsequently been published.[15]

This announcement set off a firestorm in the press. In an article on January 17, 2008 the *New York Times* proclaimed "cholesterol as a danger has its skeptics" and "cholesterol as a danger is being reassessed." [16] *Business Week* ran a major story[17] asking "Do Cholesterol Drugs Do Any Good?" The thrust of this article was the following: "Research suggests that, except among high-risk heart patients, the benefits of statins such as Lipitor are overstated."

Amazingly, the results of a single study in a small subset of patients with a rare condition called into question hundreds of studies carried out using many different medicines over decades of research. A commentary[18] in the *Journal of the American Medical Association* by Greenland and Lloyd-Jones put it this way:

> It (ENHANCE) has proved an opportunity for much misinformation to circulate in the public media including articles questioning the entire validity of cholesterol lowering despite overwhelming evidence to support the concept as a cornerstone of cardiovascular disease prevention.

So why didn't the patients on Vytorin in the ENHANCE trial have a reduction in carotid artery intima wall thickness despite having a greater reduction in LDL cholesterol? No obvious answer currently exists. It could be that the extra LDL cholesterol lowering that results from adding a cholesterol absorption inhibitor to a statin has no effect on slowing or reversing artery thickness. It could be that this patient group, which had been on multiple years of statin therapy, had already experienced the maximum benefits on the artery wall. Regardless of what occurred in this study, the ultimate answer as to whether Vytorin adds benefit over statin therapy alone won't be answered until the results of the long-term cardiovascular outcome study (IMPROVE-IT) are made available in 2011.

ENHANCE was a surrogate marker trial that did little to teach the world anything new about preventing heart attacks. One could question, as Greenland and Lloyd-Jones have done, why the sponsors chose to run such a study. However, for the press to challenge a key part of current treatment paradigms for heart disease borders on irresponsibility. By calling into question the cholesterol hypothesis, one wonders how much damage has been done. Will patients not fill prescriptions given to them by their physicians because they feel that concerns about high LDL cholesterol are overblown? Will patients stop their medications because they feel that they are not getting any protection from them?

Ironically, this controversy is coming at a time when health care providers should be reveling in the progress that has been made in reducing deaths due to cardiovascular disease. Data compiled by the American Heart Association (Figure 1.1) shows that annual increases in cardiovascular deaths that were seen for the greater part of the twentieth century have been reversed in the last 25 years. This reversal can be attributed to a number of factors: improved diagnosis and treatment, better understanding of risk factors thanks to the Framingham Study, reductions in smoking, people watching their diets and exercising more, and so on. But it would be foolish to ignore the benefits that cholesterol-lowering drugs, particularly statins, have made in this great medical story.

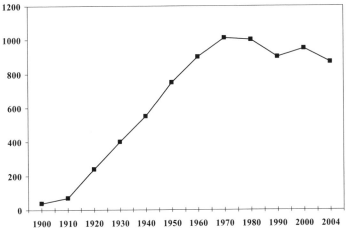

Figure 1.1   Deaths from cardiovascular disease in thousands, United States 1900–2004.

However, it is entirely possible that the progress made in lowering deaths due to cardiovascular disease will be minimized and maybe even reversed in the coming decades. The reason for this is the growing obesity epidemic that is occurring in the Western world, particularly in the United States. Epidemiology studies have shown that increased obesity in any population leads to an increase in type 2 diabetes. This, in turn, leads to an increase in deaths due to heart attacks and strokes. Unfortunately, obesity is growing at an alarming rate in the United States. The Center for Disease Control has been collecting data for obesity trends since 1985 using the Behavioral Risk Factor Surveillance System (BRFSS).[19] Obesity is defined as those people with a body mass index (BMI) of 30 or higher. To put this into perspective, a person who stands 5 feet 4 inches with a BMI of 30 would weigh 175 pounds. These data are collected from each state on an annual basis through a series of monthly telephone interviews with U.S. adults. The results from the BRFSS are jarring. In 1990, no state had an obesity prevalence of 15% or greater. The numbers were quite different in 2006, when it was found that 22 states had an obesity prevalence of greater than 25% and that two of these, Mississippi and West Virginia, had a prevalence of greater than 30% (Figure 1.2)!

As would be expected, as obesity has increased across the United States, so has diabetes. By 2005, there were 11 states that had at least 8% of their population with diabetes—a far greater prevalence than was the situation in 1994 (Figure 1.3). Cardiovascular disease increases are surely to follow.

Let's turn back to John Carey's article "Do Cholesterol Drugs Do Any Good?" Carey makes a very important point: "For anyone worried about heart disease, the first step should always be a better diet and increased physical activity. Do that, and we could cut the number of people at risk so dramatically that far fewer drugs would be needed." This is correct and everyone—physicians, health care providers, employers, and governments—should be pushing people to do this. But the fact is that

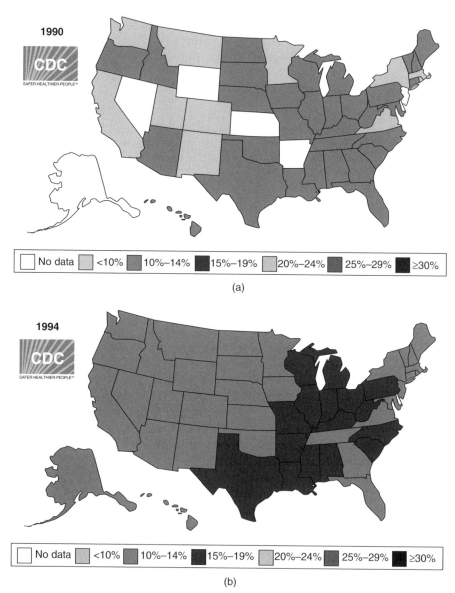

Figure 1.2   U.S. obesity prevalence: (a) 1990, (b) 1994, (c) 2006. Population with a body mass index of 30 or greater. See color insert.

effects of the obesity–diabetes–heart disease progression is going to last for decades. And this leads to a major problem in Carey's article: that only people with established heart disease should take cholesterol-lowering drugs. There is a flaw in adopting such a position. It is true that the studies which prove that reducing LDL cholesterol leads to a reduced risk of heart attacks and strokes have been done in

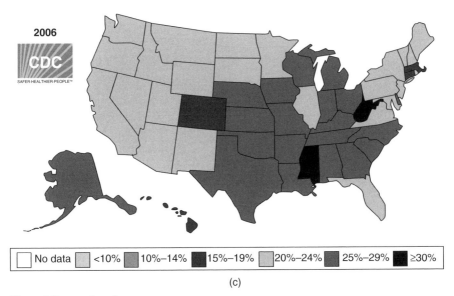

| | No data | | <10% | | 10%–14% | | 15%–19% | | 20%–24% | | 25%–29% | | ≥30% |

(c)

Figure 1.2   continued

people with documented heart disease and not in people without such documented evidence. There is a simple reason for this. Atherosclerosis is not a disease that comes on suddenly; rather, it develops over the course of decades. The long-term studies carried out with statins, despite the fact that these studies were done in people with proven disease, took as many as 5 years to complete in order to show a meaningful benefit in terms of reducing heart attacks and strokes. To show the long-term benefit of statin therapy in a young and asymptomatic population would require a decade-long trial that would be prohibitive to execute due to cost and scale. Furthermore, one might argue that the Framingham Study has already provided enough proof that reduced LDL cholesterol levels are directly related to reduced cardiovascular disease in people without documented heart disease. Finally, many people with heart disease have no symptoms until they have their first heart attack or stroke. And many times such an event is fatal. Should we be waiting for this to occur before using statins to treat people with multiple risk factors?

This brings us back to the ENHANCE trial results. Greenland and Lloyd-Jones in their *JAMA* commentary[18] make the point that "no result for the ENHANCE trial could have had any scientific or clinical importance. ..." This is because ENHANCE was not designed to measure reduction of cardiovascular events but rather to measure the effect of Vytorin on a surrogate marker, a measure of carotid artery thickness. Any meaningful clinical result for Vytorin will come from a long-term trial such as IMPROVE-IT, which measures impact of this drug on heart attacks and strokes.

It is unfortunate that the media coverage of the ENHANCE trial called into question the importance of lowering LDL cholesterol. These reports confused patients and will undoubtedly lead to fewer people taking much needed medication.

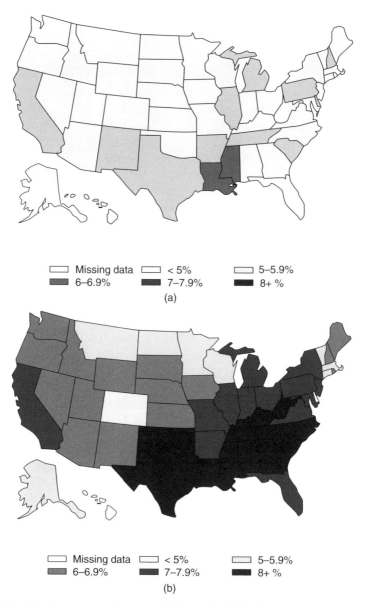

Figure 1.3   U.S. diabetes prevalence: (a) 1994 and (b) 2005. Percentage of the population with diabetes. See color insert.

Preventative medicine—be it improved diets, exercise, stopping smoking, or drugs to reduce high blood pressure and cholesterol—is critical to reducing the onslaught of cardiovascular disease that we can potentially witness in the future. Cholesterol drugs *are* necessary.

CHAPTER 2

INDUSTRY IS MORE INTERESTED IN "ME-TOO" DRUGS THAN IN INNOVATION

THE DISCOVERY and development of a new medicine is a daunting challenge. One must find a molecule that is effective against a disease, but it also must be safe. And expectations from doctors and patients are that this new drug will work in everyone for whom it is prescribed: young or old, male or female, Asian, African, European, American, and so on. Such universal utility of any medicine is unrealistic. Think about people with allergies to certain foods like peanuts or even dairy products. If there are segments of the population who cannot tolerate the staples of a normal diet, how can we expect everyone to tolerate a specific medicine equally?

Furthermore, the efficacy of medicines can differ greatly from person to person. Ask people how they treat themselves for something as simple as a headache and you hear that aspirin or ibuprofen doesn't work for them and that they need acetaminophen; or perhaps the reverse is true. The same situations arise with prescription medicines. For example, there is a class of compounds on the market to treat depression known as selective serotonin reuptake inhibitors (SSRIs). The SSRIs include such well-known drugs as Zoloft® and Paxil®. Theoretically, SSRIs should have the same effect on all patients. However, many patients for unknown reasons respond well to one SSRI but not others. Being able to choose from a range of medicines is very important for doctors to manage diseases across the broad heterogeneity of the human population.

The pharmaceutical industry is often attacked for the discovery and development of medicines referred to as "me-too" drugs.[1] A "me-too" drug is one that is structurally similar to an already known drug, but with some differences. The term "me-too" intentionally carries a negative connotation. Those who rail against "me-too" drugs believe that one entry in a new drug class should be sufficient and that the work that goes into research to generate analogous compounds is a waste of valuable resources. This is a specious argument for many reasons. First of all, as stated above, patients and physicians need options. It is highly unlikely that a single agent of a class will be safe and efficacious in all patients. Other compounds of a given class are needed.

Second, there is an implication that scientists in a company sit around and wait for a competitor's new drug to perform well on the market and then decide to get

Drug Truths: Dispelling the Myths About Pharma R&D, by John L. LaMattina
Copyright © 2009 John Wiley & Sons, Inc.

their own version. This is ludicrous. Any such strategy would be doomed to failure since, by the time the second company got through the 10- to 15-year process to bring a drug to market, the original's patent would be expired and the "me-too" would be a failure because it would be competing with low-cost generic alternatives and newer inventions.

In reality, different members of the same class of drugs result for a simple reason. Researchers from different companies attend the same scientific meetings and read the same journals. It is not unusual for people in different labs to be excited by some new insights into the cause of a disease and begin a project to discover a drug to treat it. CCR-5 antagonists and Selzentry are great examples of this. (The discovery of Selzentry will be discussed in Chapter 6.) Scientists around the world learned of the natural resistance to AIDS conferred on people by the CCR5-Δ32 mutation and then raced to get a viable CCR-5 antagonist to market. Although a number of companies sought such an agent, only Pfizer, Schering-Plough, and GlaxoSmithKline were successful in identifying compounds with the credentials to justify proceeding to late-stage development. Of these three the Pfizer entry, Selzentry, was the first to receive FDA approval. Should one of the other companies have a CCR-5 antagonist reach the marketplace, this compound would be branded by industry critics as a "me-too." Such branding would be unfair and incorrect. These programs started more than a decade ago. For the sake of AIDS patients, it was important that many efforts be made in order to bring such a new treatment to market as quickly as possible. Furthermore, having multiple CCR-5 antagonists available to patients and physicians should provide much needed options, and the ensuing competition can drive down prices. Having a second or even a third CCR-5 antagonist available would benefit people with HIV.

But most important of all is the realization that the first entry of a new class of drugs is not always the best one. Innovation often does not occur in major leaps. Rather, gradual improvements made to the original prototype are the norm. No one in their right mind would call a modern airliner a "me-too" of the Wright Brothers' Flyer. Decades of research and experimentation have led to the technological breakthroughs resulting in the aviation marvels of today. The same is true for new medicines. As good as SSRIs are in treating depression, this class of drugs is not ideal. SSRIs need to be dosed for a few weeks before they take effect. In addition, about one-third of people with depression are unaffected by SSRIs. The discovery of a modified SSRI with a rapid onset of action would be greatly appreciated by those whose lives are impacted by this disease. Unfortunately, such an agent is likely to be derided by industry critics as just another "me-too" drug.

DiMasi and Paquette of the Tufts Center for the Study of Drug Development have done an excellent analysis of the economics of follow-on (this is the term they used for "me-too") drug R&D. Their data are very enlightening.[2] They recognized that little data existed around the criticisms that follow-on drugs offer very little or no additional value. To understand this situation, they analyzed the number of first-in-class drugs introduced from 1960–1998 along with the follow-on drugs approved in the United States through 2003. In this period, 72 new therapeutic classes were introduced; from these, another 235 follow-on drugs were approved. The number of drugs per class ranged from 2 to 16, but the median was 3 and 69% of the drug classes had 4 or fewer compounds in them.

Of these 72 first-in-class drugs, 80% of them had received a priority review by the FDA. Given that these breakthrough medicines are already on the market, one would assume that a follow-on would be of little value. One might also assume that the FDA would have minimal interest in a follow-on as compared to a breakthrough drug. Actually, DiMasi and Paquette found that one-third of follow-on drugs received a priority review from the FDA. The reason for this is simple: a breakthrough first-in-class drug is not always the best-in-class.

They had other findings of interest as well.

1. Competition in the pharmaceutical industry is so fierce that nearly all classes of first-in-class drugs had at least one follow-on drug in Phase 3 testing before the first-in-class agent was approved. This supports the views that most discovery programs start at similar times.

2. Approximately one-third of first-in-class drugs to reach the U.S. market in the 1990s were *not* the first entrant of that class to enter clinical development— another indication of the intense competition that exists.

3. Multiple drugs in a class generate price competition. Of the 20 new entrants to existing classes that were introduced from 1995 to 1999, 80% were launched at a discount to the price leader.

Clearly, follow-on or "me-too" drugs provide value to patients in terms of efficacy and cost.

Perhaps the value of so-called "me-too" drugs can be described using the most successful and, arguably, one of the most important medicines ever developed, Lipitor. As measured by annual sales, Lipitor is the most successful drug in the history of the industry. It was the fifth statin to be marketed but, as outlined below, it has changed medical practice in terms of treating patients at risk for heart attacks and stroke. Yet in many ways, Lipitor can proudly claim to be a "me-too" drug.

THE FIRST STATINS

Before the advent of statins, few people had even heard the term LDL cholesterol, nor were people aware of their total cholesterol levels. However, the findings of the Framingham Heart Study coupled with the clinical benefits seen with Mevacor changed this dramatically in the late 1980s.

Not surprisingly, many companies were actively seeking HMG-CoA reductase inhibitors in the early 1980s. As we have seen, Merck launched Mevacor® in 1987 and followed-up with a superior statin, Zocor®, in 1991. Bristol-Myers Squibb launched Pravacol® also in 1991, and Sandoz (now part of Novartis) launched Lescol® in 1994. Because of the crowded marketplace at the time of the launch of Lescol, Sandoz launched it at a reduced price compared to that of the other statins—a positive resulting from a competitive marketplace. By the early 1990s, patients had four different statins to choose from. Depending on the doses given and the response of patients, a physician was now able to lower LDL cholesterol by 20–35% using one of these statins. One would have thought this would end the need for any more.

Merck was clearly a leader in the statin field and other companies were seeking HMG-CoA reductase inhibitors in the 1980s as well. An exception was Pfizer. It would be unthinkable in 2008 for a company of Pfizer's size and stature not to be in the middle of such a major research area. But the Pfizer of the mid-1980s was quite different from the company it is today. The R&D budget for all of Pfizer in 1985 was barely $300 million, and this was not only for its pharmaceutical business but also for the other businesses it had at that time such as Animal Health, Consumer Health, Chemicals, and so on. With its relatively modest R&D budget, Pfizer R&D was extremely circumspect with regard to where it invested its R&D funds. In the early 1980s, Pfizer's focus in cardiovascular research was primarily in looking for agents to treat high blood pressure. The importance of lowering blood pressure to prevent heart attacks and strokes was well established at that time and so this focus was understandable. Furthermore, Pfizer's research in the area of hypertension led to two important medicines: the calcium channel blocker, Norvasc, and the alpha blocker, Cardura.

Internal proposals were written in the 1980s to generate funding to begin an atherosclerosis research group. However, these were not originally funded. For one thing, resources were pretty tight and were needed to focus on the hypertension programs. But there was also some question as to how successful lipid-lowering drugs would actually be. At the time, it was believed that diet and exercise could be just as effective as cholestyramine and less expensive. In addition, unlike measuring blood pressure, which is easily done in a physician's office, monitoring the effects of a lipid-lowering drug requires blood tests, which are a more involved process. Finally, people were questioned whether a person who felt fine would take a medicine for decades to prevent a heart attack that might never happen anyway. Thus, Pfizer stayed on the sidelines for the statin contest.

Of course, this was a decade before Lipitor.

LIPITOR®

It is difficult for someone like me to write a section on Lipitor without having it sound like an advertisement. For one thing, I have been taking 10 mg of Lipitor daily for the last 10 years and so I can personally vouch for its effectiveness. But I have also witnessed its growth to become the biggest selling drug of all time—a position quite justified as you will see in the following pages.

Warner Lambert was one of the companies seeking an HMG-CoA reductase inhibitor in this time frame as well. Unfortunately, their research unit, Parke-Davis R&D, ran into a number of roadblocks while executing its statin program. It wasn't until late 1989 that they found a statin, code named CI-981, suitable for consideration for advancement into clinical trials. However, CI-981 would at best be the fifth statin to reach the market. More concerning was the fact that animal studies did not distinguish CI-981 from other statins.

Parke-Davis management had strong reservations about advancing CI-981 into clinical development. Given the remaining R&D investments needed to bring CI-981 to market, along with the high promotional investments that would be needed to launch this drug into a competitive marketplace of multiple established agents, the chances of this seemingly undifferentiated statin ever recouping such investments appeared to be remote. A meeting of the Parke-Davis Pharmaceutical Review Board (PRB) was held in early 1990 to determine the fate of CI-981. Going into this meeting, the sense of the PRB was to kill the program. However, a key presentation was made at this meeting by Dr. Roger Newton, the head of Atherosclerosis Biology. Roger believed strongly in CI-981 based on some of his laboratory experiments, and he felt that this compound could be more effective in humans than it had been in animals. At the end of what has now become a legendary speech, Roger got on one knee and begged the PRB to do a Phase 1 study to determine if CI-981 really could be superior to existing statins. After all, having come this far over 8 years, Roger asked the PRB why not run a final test in humans? Impressed by Roger's passion and his scientific arguments, the PRB agreed to proceed to Phase 1—a decision that eventually altered the paradigm for treating cardiovascular disease. In the multiple dose Phase 1 studies, a dose of 10 mg of CI-981 lowered LDL cholesterol by about 35%—as good as the maximum doses of the marketed statins. At a dose of 80 mg, volunteers saw their LDL cholesterol decline by nearly 60%—an unprecedented drop! Clearly, this was a drug that could be distinguished from the rest by its ability to drive down LDL cholesterol levels far more than any known agent. CI-981 was eventually given the generic name of atorvastatin and the trade name, Lipitor. Little did the people at the PRB meeting realize that, thanks to Roger Newton's plea, they had endorsed what would become the biggest selling drug of all time.

Amid all the clamor of the real value of "me-too" drugs, Parke-Davis ran a study very early in the development program which showed the importance of the greater lipid-lowering effects of Lipitor. There is a generic disease called familial hypercholesterolemia (FH) in which the homozygous form (inability of the liver to synthesize LDL receptors) results in total cholesterol levels on the order of 1000 mg/dL. As compared to the heterozygous form of FH that was described in Chapter 1, this form of FH has a prevalence of about 1 in 250,000. This degree of severity results in children having premature heart disease resulting in early death. The first marketed statins are not effective in lowering total cholesterol in these patients. In contrast, Lipitor lowered LDL cholesterol on the order of 20% in these patients. Lowering LDL from 1000 to 800 mg/dL may not seem like a major break-through, but it was for these patients. Because of their condition, these patients must undergo a process known as LDL aphaeresis. This process involves removal of a patient's blood, separation of LDL from the blood, then transfusion back into the patient. This intricate process costs about $2500. By treating these patients with 80 mg of Lipitor, the need for LDL aphaeresis sessions drops by 40%, resulting in significant annual cost savings in treating these patients and reducing the need for an uncomfortable procedure.[3]

The perspective of Dr. David Canter, who led the Lipitor development program, provides a sense of the excitement that started to build in this program.

When we started the study in homozygous FH patients, it was important at several levels. The patients were all so young and many already had severe heart disease. Would atorvastatin work? Would this be our first trial where we didn't see a good response? We had come to believe that atorvastatin was really quite different from other drugs in this class, yet how could we prove this? At another level, if the results were impressive, it would be important for accelerating the FDA review. When the results of the first four patients arrived, we knew we had something special, and so did the FDA. They gave us a Treatment IND (Investigational New Drug) based on these data three weeks later. We added an additional forty patients to the study and based on this, atorvastatin received an accelerated NDA review. Atorvastatin wasn't a cure for these patients, but it provided something extra to help them.

The results for homozygous FH showed that Lipitor fulfilled an important medical need. But this is in a small, specialized population. Does the extra LDL-lowering ability of Lipitor really provide meaningful medical value to patients with heart disease? With the launch of Lipitor in 1997, studies were initiated to answer this question. These studies were conducted by Warner-Lambert and their marketing partner, Pfizer. Pfizer continued this work once these two companies merged in 2000. Over the past 12 years, many studies have been carried out to show the importance of Lipitor in lowering cardiovascular risk across a variety of different patient populations. It is not generally appreciated that even after a drug has been approved, a company will carry out further clinical studies. Sometimes these studies, referred to as Phase 4 studies, are required by the FDA in order to gain additional safety and efficacy data for a new drug. More often, however, a company will run Phase 4 studies to demonstrate more fully the value that the new medicine brings to the health care system.

Since its launch in 1997, Pfizer has invested over $800 million in dozens of additional Lipitor studies, involving over 50,000 patients. These programs tend to be expensive to carry out because they are outcome studies designed to look at relatively large groups of patients to investigate the long-term benefits of Lipitor on improved patient survival. If successful, such studies can literally change the practice of medicine. This has, in fact, been the result of a number of these Phase 4 Lipitor studies. Three examples will be used to demonstrate this: the "Treating to New Targets" (TNT) trial, the "Collaborative Atorvastatin Diabetes Study" (CARDS), and the "Prevention of coronary and stroke events with atorvastatin in hypertensive patients who have average or lower-than-average cholesterol concentrations, in the Anglo-Scandinavian Cardiac Outcomes Trial—Lipid Lowering Arm (ASCOT-LLA): A multicentre randomised controlled trial." All of these trials were sponsored by Pfizer. These examples have been selected since each provided a better understanding for reducing heart disease in different patient populations and demonstrates that, despite being the fifth statin to reach the marketplace, Lipitor is a very important medicine.

TNT

As more has been learned about the dangers of high LDL cholesterol, guidelines as to how low a person's level should be, especially in patients who have coronary heart disease, have continued to drop. The basis for such recommendations comes

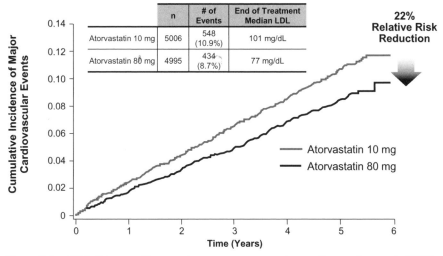

	n	# of Events	End of Treatment Median LDL
Atorvastatin 10 mg	5006	548 (10.9%)	101 mg/dL
Atorvastatin 80 mg	4995	434 (8.7%)	77 mg/dL

Figure 2.1   TNT: Primary efficacy outcome measure—major cardiovascular events (CHD death, nonfatal non-procedure-related MI, resuscitated cardiac arrest, fatal or nonfatal stroke).

from studies such as TNT. The design of TNT was quite simple. Ten thousand patients with stable coronary artery disease and with a baseline level of LDL cholesterol of less than 130 were randomly assigned in a double-blind fashion to take either 10 mg or 80 mg of Lipitor. These patients were then followed for nearly 5 years. The mean LDL cholesterol levels were 77 mg/dL for 80 mg cohort and 101 mg/dL for the 10 mg cohort. The beauty of this study is that all other parameters for patients were held constant. The only variable was the Lipitor dose and the resulting difference in LDL cholesterol levels.

The results of this study were quite remarkable. Those patients on the 80 mg dose of Lipitor had 22% fewer cardiovascular events including death due to coronary heart disease, nonfatal heart attacks, and resuscitated cardiac arrest. In addition, the 80 mg cohort had 25% fewer fatal and nonfatal strokes.[4] Simply put, lowering the LDL of these patients with the higher dose of Lipitor by 24 mg/dL had life-saving benefits (Figure 2.1).

This was a landmark trial in that, when it comes to LDL cholesterol, TNT helped to prove that "lower is better." Lipitor may have been the fifth statin to the marketplace, but its potency advantage translated in major life-saving benefits over the previous entries for patients at risk for heart attacks and strokes.

CARDS

Most of the Phase 4 work with Lipitor focused on (a) either patients with documented heart disease or (b) others who were at risk for heart disease and stroke. There are people, however, who do not have documented heart disease and do not have unusually high LDL cholesterol but who still have an increased risk of coronary vascular disease. One such population is that of type 2 diabetics. These people have two- to fourfold increased risk of both heart attack and stroke. However, in the 1990s, type 2 diabetics were not routinely prescribed lipid-lowering therapy because there was no proof that such treatment afforded any benefit to this patient population. This changed with the Collaborative Atorvastatin Diabetes Study (CARDS).[5]

CARDS was designed as a 6-year study and included 2838 patients aged 40–75 years who were randomized to placebo or 10 mg of Lipitor. These patients had no previous history of heart disease. The primary endpoint for CARDS was the first occurrence of the following: acute coronary heart disease events, coronary revascularization or stroke. The aim of the study was pretty simple: to determine whether 10 mg of Lipitor daily versus placebo reduced coronary events.

The baseline characteristics for each group were virtually identical for the Lipitor and placebo groups (an essential feature for these studies), with the average LDL levels for each being 119 and 118 mg/dL, respectively. The study, originally intended to last for 6 years, was halted 2 years early by the Data Safety Monitoring Board because one of the two groups was seeing robust reduction in coronary vascular events. Upon "unbreaking the blind" (determining which group was on drug and which was on placebo), it was found that the Lipitor group had a 35% reduction in acute coronary heart disease events, 31% fewer coronary revascularizations, and a 48% reduction in stroke. Lipitor reduced the death rate by 27%. No excess of unwanted side effects were noted in the Lipitor group; essentially, 10 mg of Lipitor had no added side effects as compared to placebo (Figure 2.2).

At the end of 4 years, the LDL levels of those patients on placebo were 122 mg/dL. However, 10 mg of Lipitor had reduced LDL cholesterol in these patients to 82 mg/dL, a third less than the placebo group. Meaningful drops in other lipid

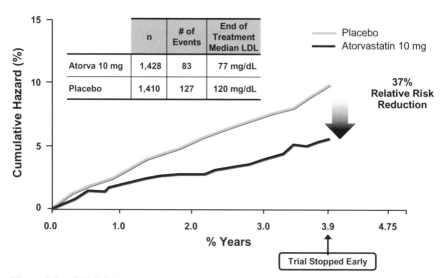

Figure 2.2 CARDS: Primary end point—major CV events (acute coronary heart disease events, coronary revascularization, or stroke).

parameters such as total cholesterol and triglycerides were also observed. These changes undoubtedly led to the enhanced protection from coronary vascular diseases that these type 2 diabetics received from Lipitor. The authors concluded their article with the following powerful statement:

> The debate about whether all patients with type 2 diabetes warrant statin treatment should now focus on whether any patients can reliably be identified as being at sufficiently low risk for this safe and efficacious treatment to be withheld.

ASCOT-LLA

The benefits of statin therapy in treating heart disease were obvious by the late 1990s. Large-scale studies with drugs like Lipitor showed the benefits of these drugs in reducing fatal and nonfatal cardiovascular events. Observational data suggested that when a number of risk factors coexisted in patients such as hypertension and high LDL cholesterol, the impact of each risk factor was enhanced. Before ASCOT, however, no study had looked at whether lowering LDL cholesterol in patients with high blood pressure who had moderate or lower lipid levels would benefit from statin treatment.

ASCOT was a study that looked at the long-term benefits of two different blood pressure medications in lowering heart disease. This trial, however, had a lipid-lowering arm (LLA) as part of the study.[6] Those patients with total cholesterol of 250 mg/dL or lower were randomized to receive either 10 mg of Lipitor (atorvastatin) or a placebo along with their blood pressure medication. In all, there were 10,305 patients in the LLA. The study was scheduled to run for 5 years, which was deemed the length of time needed to see a meaningful effect on reducing heart attacks and strokes.

ASCOT was conceived, designed, and coordinated not by Pfizer but by an investigator-led independent steering committee. The results were reviewed on a monthly basis by an independent Data Safety Monitoring Board (DSMB). Despite the fact that the trial was supposed to continue for 5 years, the DSMB halted the trial after a little over 3 years on the grounds that those in the Lipitor arm had a highly significant reduction in nonfatal heart attacks and fatal cardiac events compared with those on placebo. There were 89 cases of fatal and nonfatal stroke on Lipitor compared to 121 on placebo. In terms of total cardiovascular events, 389 occurred on Lipitor versus 486 on placebo. Figure 2.3 depicts these results and shows that the beneficial effect with Lipitor is seen in the early stages of this trial.

Despite the fact that these patients were considered to be moderate to low with respect to their cholesterol levels, the benefits of reducing their cholesterol cannot be questioned.

The authors ended their publication with the following:

> Our findings in the ASCOT lipid-lowering arm show important and large relative reductions in cardiovascular events associated with the use of atorvastatin 10 mg among a population of hypertensive patients who on average were, despite other risk factors,

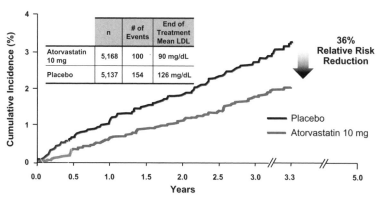

Figure 2.3   ASCOT-LLA primary endpoint: Nonfatal MI and fatal CHD.

at only moderate cardiovascular risk and who would not conventionally have been deemed dyslipidaemic. We hope our results will help to close the gap between what is recommended and the current suboptimal use of lipid-lowering treatment in clinical practice.

The Lipitor story is instructive on a number of fronts. The first statins proved to be important medicines. But Lipitor brought a higher degree of cholesterol lowering that enabled the full potential of this class of compounds to be fully appreciated. Furthermore, some studies have suggested that Lipitor has other beneficial properties, known as pleiotropic effects, which result in protection of the vasculature to a far greater extent than would be expected from the lipid changes alone.[7,8] Most important, however, have been the results from the post-approval studies for Lipitor. These have literally changed medical practice. Patients with diabetes are now included in the high-risk category in terms of the treatment of LDL cholesterol. Patients with hypertension are recommended to take statins even if their LDL cholesterol appears to be in a moderate range. Finally, while the recommended LDL cholesterol goal for patients at high risk for heart attack and stroke is <100 mg/dL, when the risk is very high, LDL cholesterol levels of 70 mg/dL are called for.[9]

These changes in medical practice have all resulted from Roger Newton's plea to senior leaders at Parke-Davis to study a so-called "me-too" drug. Thankfully, for the benefit of the millions of heart patients, they said yes.

CHAPTER 3

IT TAKES INDUSTRY TOO LONG TO DISCOVER NEW DRUGS

I**F A** scientist has a novel idea today for a cure to Alzheimer's Disease and if he or she worked in an environment where this idea can be prosecuted with alacrity, it would still take at least 9–10 years for that idea to reach patients as an approved medicine. And that is assuming everything goes well and minimal roadblocks are encountered. The process for discovering and developing a new medicine is incredibly difficult and complex. The former CEO of GlaxoSmithKline, Jean-Pierre Garnier, once said it is more difficult to discover and develop a new medicine than it is to put a man on the moon. This is not an exaggeration.

The process begins when a scientist, seeking an approach to treat a disease where a medical need exists, is stimulated to pursue a particular avenue of research. The stimulation can come from a variety of sources. Perhaps the scientist has heard a lecture or read a paper that sparks an idea on a project he or she would like to pursue. Perhaps he or she has heard about certain progress made by a competitor which can be improved upon. Regardless of the source, the scientist will set in motion a number of experiments which will build in time to hundreds of people working together to convert this early idea into a valued medicine. The overall process can be broken down into five distinct stages.

1. *Candidate Identification.* This is the early experimentation that leads to a compound which has the potential to enter clinical trials. This phase is often called "discovery" and is focused on inventing a compound that has the credentials to justify its worthiness for clinical studies. This generally takes 3–5 years.

2. *Preclinical Studies.* Once an interesting compound is in hand, a number of tests are required to demonstrate its safety in animals, its stability, its body distribution and metabolism, and so on. It is not unusual for a compound to fail one of these tests, thereby ending this compound's progress. The project team will then move back into the discovery phase in order to find a replacement for the discontinued prototype. Overall, the successful completion of these preclinical studies results in the filing of an IND (Investigational New Drug) with the FDA. If the FDA deems that the package meets the necessary safety and efficacy hurdles, it will permit clinical studies to begin. In general, this preclinical phase takes 12 months to complete.

Drug Truths: Dispelling the Myths About Pharma R&D, by John L. LaMattina
Copyright © 2009 John Wiley & Sons, Inc.

3. *Phase 1.* The first step in the clinic involves testing the compound in healthy volunteers, first as single doses in increasing increments followed by multiple doses ultimately in the range where human activity is anticipated. This is done to find an efficacious dose of the drug that can be safely tested. In the majority of cases, Phase 1 studies simply show that the compound is safe and well-tolerated. These studies do not determine if the compound works against the disease for which it is targeted. However, sometimes one can obtain information of the impact of the experimental medicine on a surrogate marker such as the lowering of blood pressure, a marker for heart disease, or decreasing plasma glucose, a marker for diabetes. It takes about 12 months to gather and interpret these data.

4. *Phase 2.* Once the effects of a drug are tested and it is deemed safe in healthy volunteers, it is then moved into trials in people who have the condition being treated to determine if the experimental medicine does mitigate the disease. Depending on the nature of the disease, this is the most important step in the whole drug discovery and development process because a strong efficacy signal needs to be seen to justify further advancement. Phase 2 studies also attempt to find the right dose for the drug, determine how often to give the drug, and identify which patients can benefit from this potential new medicine. It can take 12–30 months to measure the experimental medicine's effects adequately.

5. *Phase 3.* If the Phase 2 trial has positive results, the experimental medicine moves into large-scale clinical trials designed to demonstrate safety and efficacy in patents over a much longer period of time. The new drug is tested side-by-side with an approved existing therapy and placebo, or, if no therapy exists, it is tested only against a placebo. The length and size of these trials are dependent on whether the drug is intended for acute use (for example, treating an infectious disease) or for chronic use (to treat diabetes) because the latter situation calls for long-term studies. Thus, Phase 3 studies can take 2–5 years, depending on the intended use of a drug.

Finally, upon successful completion of these steps, a company will file a New Drug Application (NDA) with regulatory agencies around the world. The amount of information contained in an NDA is mind-boggling. In the days before electronic data filing, it literally took trucks to deliver these materials to the FDA. Picture a room 16×16 feet filled from floor to ceiling with scientific documents and you get a sense of the size of an NDA. It is no wonder that this review usually takes a year. Sometimes the first action taken by the FDA on the NDA is an approval. Oftentimes, however, the submitter of the NDA is asked to provide clarifications or even carry out additional studies so the approval process can take longer. And in many cases, the FDA will call in an expert Advisory Committee made up of key scientists to offer guidance and recommendations about the proposed new medicine before rendering a final decision.

The overall process from idea to product can therefore take from 9 to 16+ years to complete. Furthermore, historically only one in 20 compounds that start the development process ever become marketed drugs. This is not an enterprise for people with a low tolerance for failure or for those who need immediate gratification. The great majority of researchers will never see the fruits of their labor result in a new medication in the marketplace.

The above description is greatly simplified, and it does not necessarily capture the rollercoaster nature of the process. The best way to teach this is with a specific example, and this will be done with the story of torcetrapib.

ANOTHER SCIENTIFIC CONTROVERSY

As has been outlined in Chapters 1 and 2, great strides have been made in the last 20 years in the reduction of deaths due to cardiovascular diseases. This is due to a variety of factors such as better treatments, improved detection of early disease and lifestyle changes. But there is no doubt that one of the most significant pharmaceutical breakthroughs in the battle against heart disease has been the advent of the class of drugs knows as statins. Even with the advent of statins, however, almost a million deaths in the United States still occur each year due to cardiovascular disease, with the estimated direct and indirect costs amounting to $393 billion in 2005.[1] As effective as statins are, long-term clinical studies have shown they reduce cardiovascular risk by about 35%. To put this into perspective, over the next 4-year period, if 100 patients with cardiovascular disease would have suffered a heart attack or stroke without Lipitor, only 65 would have suffered a heart attack or stroke had they taken the medication. The obvious question that this raises is, how can cardiovascular disease be further reduced beyond the success of statins?

Perhaps the answer lies in Figure 3.1, which is taken from the landmark Framingham Heart Study[2] which was described earlier. This chart shows the importance of not just LDL cholesterol levels but also HDL cholesterol levels in mitigating the risk of a heart attack over a 4-year period. HDL (high-density lipoprotein) cholesterol is known as the "good" cholesterol. High HDL cholesterol levels are known to be "cardio protective," although the exact mechanism of this protection is not

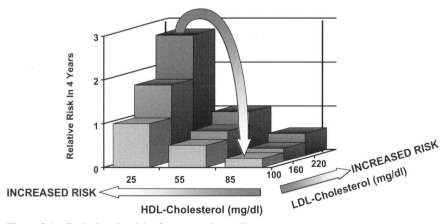

Figure 3.1   Reducing the risk of coronary heart disease.

absolutely defined. HDL cholesterol is known to be involved in "reverse cholesterol transport," a process whereby cholesterol is removed from coronary vessels and cleared through the liver. HDL cholesterol also appears to have anti-inflammatory properties and anti-thrombotic properties, and it prevents the formation of "oxidized-LDL" a form of "bad" cholesterol that builds up rapidly in artery walls. HDL cholesterol also decreases the ability of "adhesion molecules" to damage arterial walls, which is the start of atherogenesis. All of these activities could contribute to the beneficial effects of high HDL cholesterol levels.

The Framingham Study shows that, while lowering LDL cholesterol can reduce cardiovascular risk, increasing HDL cholesterol might reduce cardiovascular risk even more dramatically. Unfortunately, raising HDL cholesterol significantly is not an easy thing to do. Distance running and red wine are known to increase HDL cholesterol, but only modestly. Niacin can increase HDL cholesterol by 15–20%, but it has unwelcomed side effects. For one thing, it causes uncomfortable flushing. I personally have experienced this effect. Before becoming a Lipitor devotee, I tried slow-release niacin to control my dyslipidemia. Unfortunately, the flushing that occurred unexpectedly at various times of the day caused me to stop taking it. Beyond the flushing, niacin can harm the liver and can also raise blood sugar.

Thus, an objective and well-tolerated agent that raised HDL cholesterol was needed. As often happens in science, one knows where to go, the question is how do you get there?

THE SPARK

In late 1990 the *New England Journal of Medicine*[3] published a study that prompted 17 years of research at Pfizer and other companies. This article, "Increased High-Density Lipoprotein Levels Caused by a Common Cholesteryl-Ester Transfer Protein Gene Mutation," described a cholesteryl-ester transfer protein (CETP) gene mutation in four families from three different regions of Japan. These family members who completely lacked CETP had markedly increased levels of HDL cholesterol and decreased levels of LDL cholesterol. More importantly, there was no evidence of premature atherosclerosis (commonly called "hardening of the arteries") in families with this CETP deficiency. The authors concluded with the following statement: "In fact, the lipoprotein profile of persons with CETP deficiency is potentially anti-atherogenic and may be associated with an increased life span."

This study provided the clue needed to hunt for a way to raise HDL cholesterol. Theoretically, if a compound could be developed which inhibited CETP inside the body, one could pharmacologically mimic the genetic gift that prevented the synthesis of CETP in those Japanese families. By inhibiting CETP in people predisposed to heart disease, one might be able to reduce the risk of a heart attack dramatically, thereby improving upon the benefits that had already been seen with statins.

However, experts in the field of atherosclerosis disagreed about the potential benefits of raising HDL cholesterol by CETP inhibition. Some worried that complete CETP inhibition could cause the accumulation of very large dysfunctional HDL cholesterol and abnormal LDL cholesterol. Others questioned the wisdom of interfering with normal cholesterol transport pathways, and the long-term impact of doing this could be negative.

Again, we have the dilemma often found in medical science. A promising and intriguing hypothesis exists and generates heated debates. However, the only way to answer the key question is to invent a compound that can then be used to test the hypothesis in people. This is the essential contribution that the pharmaceutical industry makes to advance medical science. *Only pharmaceutical R&D discovers, develops, manufactures, tests, and demonstrates the properties of compounds that prove or disprove medical hypotheses.* Nowhere else is this done.

FINDING TORCETRAPIB

In 1991 when I was leading the chemistry efforts of Pfizer's Metabolic Diseases research, we began a program to find a potent CETP inhibitor. This proved to be extremely challenging. CETP is a large protein, and oftentimes finding a small molecule to inhibit the function of such a protein is nearly impossible. Why is a small molecule important? For treating a chronic condition like heart disease, it is helpful for a patient to be able to take a pill daily. Small molecules can be easily absorbed and can readily be made into oral therapy. Large molecules, however, do not survive in the gut and so they must be administered as infusions. For almost 3 years, Pfizer scientists looked for such a molecule. Hundreds of thousands of molecules were screened and tested against the protein. In addition, many compounds were newly synthesized and tested as well. Unfortunately, none had the type of activity we were seeking.

At this point the project was close to being discontinued. The CETP hypothesis was promising, but further pursuit of it was useless without a compound to test it. However, a young chemist, Dr. Roger Ruggeri, was assigned the task of checking on some final possibilities. In doing so, he hit upon a small molecule compound that weakly bound to CETP. Over the following weeks and months, he synthesized analogs (modified versions) of this initial lead structure trying to boost its activity altering the physical chemical properties of the compounds, thereby helping them to bind better to CETP. In doing so, Roger improved the binding of these molecules to CETP by 100-fold.

These modifications made the compounds active when tested *in vitro* (essentially in a test tube). However, these same modifications made the compounds unsuitable for testing in animals since they were "greasy" and virtually insoluble. This lack of solubility made these compounds impossible to absorb from the gut when given orally. A biologist on the project, Mr. Ron Clark, in trying to facilitate *in vivo* testing, decided to dissolve the compounds in olive oil. This simple change made all the difference. Subsequent animal testing showed that these inhibitors of CETP provided unprecedented increases in HDL cholesterol. When Ron had gotten the first exciting results from the animal studies, he left them on the desk of the program's leader, Dr. Mark Bamberger. Mark was away at a scientific meeting when the results were generated. When Mark returned and saw the data, he initially thought it was a prank—it was April Fool's Day. However, the results were quite real. Suddenly, this program got very interesting!

The identification of a biologically active molecule is a key milestone. But this is far from having a compound ready for clinical trials. First, scientists need to maximize the intrinsic activity of the compound. Also some fundamental studies are needed to understand how and what happens to the compound inside the body, if it may have negative interactions with other drugs, how safe it is in early animal studies, how stable it is, and so on. This is often painstaking work in that each modification made to a molecule can alter a number of these parameters and not necessarily in a favorable manner. In the CETP program, it took about two and a half years to go from Roger's first active compound to an experimental medicine suitable for testing in humans. This compound was code named CP-529,414 and was later given the generic name torcetrapib. In September 1997, after more than 6 years of laborious lab work, this compound was approved by the early development management team for extensive animal safety studies necessary in preparation for human testing.

Despite the progress made to this point, having a viable formulation to use in the clinic was still an issue. While olive oil worked well in the laboratory, a more practical presentation of torcetrapib was needed. Such challenges are addressed by a group within Pfizer called Pharmaceutical Sciences. This group has a wide range of responsibilities including: devising large-scale syntheses of experimental medicines, determining how stable these are, and devising the best delivery methods for potential new drugs. They tested a number of different technologies, but they all proved problematic. However, working in collaboration with Bend Research in Oregon, a major breakthrough was made using a method now known as "spray-dried dispersion" (SDD). SDD means dissolving the insoluble drug and a polymer (hydroxy propyl methyl cellulose acetate succinate—HPMCAS) in an organic solvent and then spray-drying this solution. The resultant molecular dispersion is very stable (meaning the drug can be stored) and, more importantly, can be easily absorbed into the bloodstream. The SDD formulation of torcetrapib improved its solubility 100-fold, thereby enabling the first studies in humans to begin. The Bend scientists did a great job in developing this methodology, a first in the industry.

PHASE 1 / 2 CLINICAL STUDIES

The first volunteers received torcetrapib in August 1999. For many drugs, Phase 1 studies are simply designed to measure safety and metabolism. It is not often that one can get a sense of whether the mechanism of action of a new drug can be proven in such an early study with healthy volunteers.

However, with torcetrapib profound effects were seen in the lipid profiles of the volunteers in this study even with single doses. The results of 14 days of torcetrapib treatment in healthy individuals are depicted in Figure 3.2.

Simply stated, torcetrapib treatment resulted in dose-related increases in HDL cholesterol and decreases in LDL cholesterol to a degree that was unprecedented—and more than had been envisioned. In general, torcetrapib was very well tolerated,

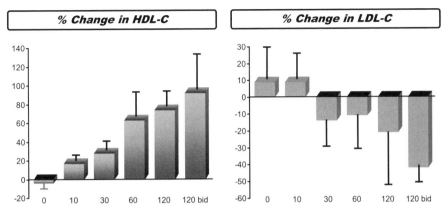

Figure 3.2   Proof of mechanism for CETP inhibition in healthy individuals. Effects on lipid profile during treatment with torcetrapib versus placebo for 14 days.

with one exception. At the high doses, blood pressure increased by about 2 mm of mercury. This resulted in the use of a dose of 60 mg of torcetrapib in subsequent studies as this lower dose did not cause blood pressure increases in Phase 1 studies in healthy volunteers.

The next step was to study torcetrapib in patients with cardiovascular disease (Phase 2). Here another surprise was uncovered. Early Phase 2 data showed that the LDL cholesterol lowering seen with torcetrapib was highly variable and, in patients with triglyceride levels in excess of 150 mg/dL, LDL cholesterol actually increased. This variance was eliminated when torcetrapib was combined with atorvastatin (the active ingredient of Lipitor), suggesting that torcetrapib could work best with background statin therapy.

This result changed the thinking around how best to run the clinical program. Going back to the Framingham Heart Study data, it is clear that the best way to minimize the risk of heart attack and stroke is to *raise* HDL cholesterol and *lower* LDL cholesterol simultaneously. Thus, combining torcetrapib with a statin made sense medically. However, running a Phase 3 program with multiple statins in combination with torcetrapib would be extremely impractical. After consulting external medical advisers, it was decided that the Phase 3 program would test a combination of torcetrapib and atorvastatin against atorvastatin alone. Why use atorvastatin? Cynics said because this is a Pfizer drug. It was irrefutable, however, that atorvastatin was both the most used and most studied drug in the history of medicine. This was easily the best choice for patients and made scientific sense.

Not everyone agreed with the decision to run the Phase 3 program in this fashion. An editorial in the *New England Journal of Medicine* made the accusation that marketing was driving the research agenda.[4a] The major concern raised in the editorial was that, by studying torcetrapib in combination with atorvastatin, a physician would only have access to this CETP inhibitor with only one statin. Should a physician want to combine torcetrapib with another statin, he or she would be out of luck. That was clearly not the case.[4b] Pfizer's plan had always been to file an NDA for torcetrapib as a stand-alone agent, provided that the CETP hypothesis was confirmed in the clinic with the torcetrapib/atorvastatin (T/A) combination.[5]

The appearance of this editorial in such a prestigious journal showed the great interest in this program. Here was a compound just starting Phase 3 clinical trials. It was years away from the marketplace. Yet, leading physicians were commenting on the clinical program. Such interest in a drug in early Phase 3 is relatively rare and attributable to the potential that torcetrapib had with respect to revolutionizing the treatment of cardiovascular disease.

Subsequent Phase 2 studies with T/A showed profound lipid remodeling, with HDL cholesterol increasing by 60% and LDL cholesterol dropping by 60%. To put this into perspective, a person who had an HDL cholesterol of 30 and an LDL cholesterol of 200, when dosed with T/A, would see their lipid profile convert to an HDL cholesterol of 48 and an LDL cholesterol of 80—a lipid profile that theoretically should greatly reduce the relative risk of coronary artery disease. These lipid results and the accumulated safety data propelled T/A to Phase 3.

PHASE 3

This stage of the drug discovery/development continuum is the most complex and costly. The investment needed depends on the nature of the disease that the new medicine is targeting. For an acute use drug, such as a novel antibiotic to treat life-threatening Methacillin-resistant *Staphylococcus aureus* (MRSA) infections, short-term clinical studies are required because the drug will only be used in patients for the time needed to clear the infection. However, a drug to prevent heart attacks and strokes will be taken by patients for the rest of their lives. Thus, long-term safety and efficacy trials are needed in Phase 3 to assure the benefits of the new medicine outweigh any risks.

In general, the investment needed in discovery to carry out all the work to identify a potential new medicine can range from $25 to $30 million. This is what it takes just to get to Phase 1. Interestingly, these early costs tend to be fairly standard because it generally takes the same number of scientists and similar resources to discover a new drug for rare diseases as it does for drugs to treat the most prevalent conditions. Similarly, Phase 1 testing also tends not to vary among new medicines and so these studies amount to $10–$15 million per compound. At Phase 2, costs vary depending on the information that is needed to justify the major Phase 3 trials. Thus, a Phase 2 program can cost between $60 and $100 million. However, all of the costs to this point are dwarfed by the ultimate Phase 3 program. Before Phase 3, perhaps as many as 500 people have been studied with the new drug. Phase 3, however, involves thousands of patients in many different complex studies and testing for periods that can last for years. The large investment in Phase 3, anywhere from $400 to $800 million, requires full approval at the highest levels of a company.

The costs for running Phase 3 clinical trials are often questioned by those not familiar with the process. These studies are run by independent physicians at hospitals around the globe. While each trial is different, there are basic work units that

---

Investigators
 - patient recruitment
 - recording clinical results
 - monitoring adverse events

Laboratories
 - full battery of blood tests

Study Monitors
 - site visits to assure accurate data collection and adverse event
   recording

Data Managers
 - accumulate data bases, check for errors and assure data consistency

Study Managers
 - assure that sites get blinded supplies of drugs
 - assure that staff at the site is properly trained

Statisticians
 - perform data analyses

Administrative Support
 - help run the studies

Data Safety Monitoring Board
 - payments for travel, meeting venues, data compilation

Figure 3.3   Basis of the costs for Phase 3 clinical trials.

must be done to execute each study. A menu of these items appears in Figure 3.3. The cost of these tasks can vary, depending on the type of clinical trial being run. As an example, it is not unusual for investigator fees to amount to $10,000 per patient for a single long-term study. For a study that involves an invasive surgical technique such as intravascular coronary artery ultrasound (IVUS), costs are significantly higher.

It should be noted that Figure 3.3 only focuses on the costs for running clinical trials. Another major expenditure involves making bulk quantities of the drug to be tested as well as obtaining sufficient quantities of the comparator drug to be used in the study. Furthermore, the drug samples need to be "blinded" in such a way that neither the doctor nor the patient knows if the drug being administered is the experimental medicine, the comparative medicine, or placebo. Depending on the nature of the clinical trials, drug supply costs can add tens of millions of dollars to a Phase 3 program.

Thus, to bring a single new medicine to market costs between $500 million and $1 billion. In fact, DiMasi and colleagues at the Tufts Center for the Study of Drug Development pegged these costs for new drug development at $802 million in 2003.[6] This is a key point. There are those who purport that clinical trials cost far less than this. A notable example is Dr. Marcia Angell, the former Editor-in-Chief of the *New England Journal of Medicine* who during an interview[7] claimed that "They give a figure of $800 million . . . it is nowhere near there. The best educated guess is that it is less than $100 million." Were that only true!

The torcetrapib/atorvastatin (T/A) Phase 3 program was expected to cost $800 million, the most expensive ever run at Pfizer and perhaps in the entire industry. Yet, until this point, all that had been demonstrated was that T/A caused dramatic improvements in a patient's HDL/LDL profile. While this was intriguing to the FDA and other regulatory agencies, these data alone would not support the approval of a New Drug Application (NDA). The long-term benefits in terms of reducing cardiovascular deaths by altering lipids via CETP inhibition were still hypothetical. Furthermore, T/A did cause a small but real increase in blood pressure. Outcome studies were still needed to demonstrate that treating patients predisposed to heart attack and stroke with T/A reduced this risk. Furthermore, this reduced risk needed to be shown to be superior to the benefits produced by atorvastatin alone. Based on the known association between HDL cholesterol, blood pressure, and cardiovascular disease, the large increase in HDL cholesterol was expected to provide much greater benefit than any harm caused in some patients by the small increase in blood pressure.

It is interesting to contrast this situation with that discussed in Chapter 1 for Vytorin and ENHANCE. While LDL cholesterol was an established surrogate marker for heart disease, that is not true today for HDL cholesterol. The FDA will not approve a drug based solely on its ability to raise HDL cholesterol. Long-term outcome studies are needed to prove that such an action results in a decrease in cardiovascular events such as fatal and nonfatal heart attacks. This difference between LDL cholesterol and HDL cholesterol as surrogate markers has recently been discussed in a commentary in the *Journal of the American Medical Association*.[8]

The full development program included 62 studies that investigated such things as the effects of T/A in patients with different lipid profiles, the impact of dosing at various times of the day, and potential drug–drug interactions because this patient population tends to require multiple medications. All of these studies are necessary in order to be able to provide a full profile of a new medicine to regulatory authorities. However, there were two major components that distinguished the T/A clinical Phase 3 program. First, there were atherosclerosis imaging studies designed to look at the thickness of artery walls using two different methods: carotid ultrasound and coronary IVUS (intravascular ultrasound). These studies had approximately 1000 patients in each, and patients were randomized to take either T/A or atorvastatin for 24 months. The goal of these studies was quite simple. If the CETP hypothesis was correct, then at the end of the study the patients on T/A should have less arterial plaque compared to patients on atorvastatin alone. Reduced plaque would be expected to reduce the risk of cardiac events.

Imaging studies are tough to execute. For example, IVUS studies involve a surgical procedure in which a catheter is inserted in the femoral artery of the groin and snaked into the heart. Patients volunteering for such studies are usually identified because they have a clinical need for such a procedure. At the tip of the catheter is a device that, via ultrasonic waves, can take very precise pictures of the arteries. Two years later, the process is repeated and the doctor can see the impact of the drug on atherosclerosis.

While these imaging studies can be enlightening, they still do not conclusively demonstrate reduced cardiovascular risk. Thus, the second distinguishing feature that underpinned the entire Phase 3 program was a study to measure morbidity and mortality (death). This study, known as ILLUMINATE (Investigation of Lipid Level Management to understand its impact IN Atherosclerotic Events), involved 15,067 patients (7533 on T/A; 7534 on atorvastatin) who were to be followed for an average of 4.5 years. If the CETP hypothesis was correct, the number of cardiovascular events seen between treatments would be significantly different in favor of the T/A group.

It is important to understand how studies like these are conducted. The sponsor company works with regulators like the FDA and investigators to design studies that meet the regulatory needs. Once the study protocols are agreed to, the sponsor invites hospitals and clinics around the world to recruit the appropriate patients for the study. At each hospital, these studies are first approved by that institution's Investigational Review Board (IRB). In a major M&M study such as ILLUMINATE, the progress of the whole study is monitored by an independent Data Safety Monitoring Board (DSMB). The DSMB is made up of independent experts in their field who follow the study closely and who meet periodically to discuss the results as they emerge. The DSMB deliberations do not include the sponsor. Rather, each month the sponsor is simply told to begin, alter, or stop the study. A study can be stopped if the results seen to date are so beneficial that all patients should be given the new medicine. Alternatively, a DSMB could stop a study because the new drug offers no benefit or because it is proving to be inferior to the standard therapy.

Often one will hear cynicism when a study describing the benefits of a new medicine appears in a medical journal. The cynicism is due to the fact that the sponsor funded the study, and so there is an assumption that the study must be biased. The sponsor does in fact fund these studies. However, the FDA reviews the protocols and IRBs ascertain that the study is ethical and can be properly carried out. The study is conducted by individual doctors with a duty to their patients, and it is overseen by an independent steering committee; clinical events are adjudicated by another independent group; and finally the results are analyzed by yet another independent statistical group, and all of this under the watchful eye of the DSMB. Each of these studies is carried out in a very high professional, unbiased, and ethical manner.

The protocols were in place, the patients were recruited, and the studies began. In a few years, the answer would be in hand.

THE RESULTS

On November 30, 2006 Pfizer held a major meeting with financial analysts and members of the press to discuss its pipeline. More than 400 people converged on the Pfizer Global Research and Development laboratories site in Groton, Connecticut for "R&D Day." Such days are held periodically to update shareholders and the general public on the progress being made by the world's largest R&D organization. Coincidentally, Pfizer's previous "R&D Day" had occurred on November 30, 2004. Given that two years had passed since the previous event, there would be a lot of review at this session.

This "R&D Day" had special meaning because it was the first for Pfizer's new CEO, Jeff Kindler. It was a chance for Jeff to show his commitment to R&D and his desire for Pfizer to be known as "the Science Company." As one might expect, a great deal of preparation went into this meeting. Pfizer felt they had a great pipeline of new medicines in early development, and they wanted to spread this enthusiasm to the rest of the world.

A host of new and exciting potential medicines were described. The latest data for Chantix, a soon-to-be-launched medicine to halt nicotine addition, was presented. A whole new approach to treat AIDS, embodied by Selzentry, was described as were new approaches to controlling pain highlighted by Lyrica, which had been found to be effective for previously difficult to treat conditions such as neuropathic pain and fibromyalgia. A revolutionary new treatment for rheumatoid arthritis was unveiled, as were new compounds to eradicate bacterial infections that were now resistant to traditional antibiotics. And if all this wasn't enough, multiple new anticancer agents were described: compounds that prevent tumors from growing blood vessels thereby starving them of nutrients; compounds that could help one's own immune system to fight the cancer; and compounds that were genetically targeted to halt tumor growth. In fact, Pfizer scientists envisioned that this portfolio of anticancer agents could eventually turn cancer into a controllable disease and perhaps even cure it. Pfizer was on the cusp of finding the "holy grail" of making cancer a disease to be no longer feared.

However, what the crowd really wanted to hear about was torcetrapib.

This compound generated unprecedented interest in the medical and financial communities because everyone recognized that, if successful, it would provide a revolutionary treatment for reducing cardiovascular disease, which was still the major cause of death globally. Given the medical and commercial success of a statin like Lipitor, the potential for T/A was great. This drug was viewed by many as potentially the next big breakthrough in treating cardiovascular disease.

From the very first reports on the efficacy of torcetrapib in clinical trials showing that this compound had unprecedented effects in remodeling a patient's lipids, torcetrapib became a focal point for any discussion about Pfizer. Any and all meetings with financial analysts had multiple questions about the torcetrapib clinical programs: How is patient recruitment going? Has the FDA agreed to approve this compound on vascular imaging data alone? Will Pfizer sell torcetrapib only in combination with atorvastatin (the active ingredient of Lipitor)? Are there side effects emerging in the clinical trials?

So, at R&D Day on November 30, 2006, Pfizer had diligently prepared for a slew of questions on torcetrapib. Furthermore, the interest was further heightened by the fact that Pfizer's competitors were beginning to announce that they too were developing their own CETP inhibitors. Thus, Pfizer braced themselves for a new set of questions as to whether these competitive compounds were superior to torcetrapib. This field of research had become the hottest in the pharmaceutical industry.

From Pfizer's perspective, R&D Day went very well. Their overall pipeline progress was well-received. Analysts and members of the press came away with a good sense of Pfizer's pipeline and the progress that had been made. And, as anticipated, torcetrapib dominated the session. But the clinical data continued to be compelling and the high caliber of research being carried out was clear to all in attendance. Confidence was running very high in this program.

All of this changed 40 hours later.

Dr. Chuck Shear was the head of the T/A clinical trials program. He was the first to get the news.

I remember waking up on that crisp Saturday morning. I was looking forward to some downtime as the project had been going 24/7 for a few years now. It was about 3 AM—my usual wakeup time—when checking through my email, there was a message from the night before that Philip Barter (chair of the T/A Data Safety Monitoring Board) needed to talk to me and that it was urgent. Been there, done that, I thought. Everything about T/A was urgent, so I waited until 6 AM knowing that Philip was even more sleep deprived than I.

"Are you sitting down?" Philip said. "You won't believe this, but the DSMB recommended terminating the trial, and I agreed with them."

"What, you're kidding!" was my reply. How could this be possible; it wasn't even a scenario we had on our radar screen. "Are you sure?" I said. "You have to see the data yourself," he replied.

In reviewing the latest ILLUMINATE trial data on the evening of December 1, 2006, the DSMB noted an imbalance of all-cause mortality in T/A compared to atorvastatin that crossed the prespecified boundary for stopping the trial. As a result, these independent experts recommended terminating the ILLUMINATE trial.

The Pfizer CEO, Jeff Kindler, was informed of this recommendation at 7 AM that Saturday morning. He was just getting ready to begin an annual rite, making his daughter her favorite breakfast—pancakes—for her birthday. Instead, Jeff immediately halted all studies with T/A and Pfizer's other CETP inhibitor in earlier development. He then called all senior leaders to Pfizer's New York City offices for an 11:00 AM meeting to discuss how best to inform patients and key leaders of this outcome. Jeff will likely think of the T/A program whenever he again makes pancakes.

By this time, the patients in the vascular imaging studies—both the carotid ultrasound studies and the intravascular ultrasound (IVUS) study—had already completed almost all of their 24-month dosing. Thus, despite the fact that patients would no longer be dosed with T/A, analyses of these studies could be completed. The results of these studies were equally surprising. Despite the 62% rise in HDL cholesterol, *no improvements* were seen with T/A over atorvastatin alone either in carotid intima-media thickness[9a-c] or in measurement of percent atheroma volume,[10] two separate measures of a patients "hardened arteries."

Experts in the field were disappointed. Dr. Steven E. Nissen, Chairman of Cardiovascular Medicine at the Cleveland Clinic and the lead investigator of the IVUS trial, perhaps said it best.[11] "These findings further demonstrate the great difficulty in developing therapies to disrupt the atherosclerotic disease process."

So what went wrong? Is the CETP hypothesis flawed? Is more complete inhibition of CETP required in order to mimic the genetic mutations seen in Japanese families? Is the torcetrapib molecule flawed and causing problems unrelated to its CETP inhibitor properties? Did the blood pressure increase seen with torcetrapib counterbalance the beneficial HDL cholesterol elevating properties? All of these questions have and will continue to be debated. However, the bottom line for this specific program is quite simple. Although T/A dramatically remodeled the lipid profile of people at risk for cardiovascular disease, it did not benefit these patients.

But what about the hundreds of scientists who saw their 17 years of work end overnight? How did they feel? Chuck Shear's poignant comments below perhaps express it best.

> I know I entered an alternate reality that day—although I don't know it to be the case—it must be something that anyone in bereavement must feel. Something was gone that would never be replaced, a hole in my heart that will remain forever. I remember on the Metro-North train traveling down to New York City that morning—it was full of little kids laughing and carrying on and going to see the tree lighting in the city that was later that day. I just couldn't grasp what had happened. My wife, Deb, said it best. I was acting as though I had lost a 6-year-old child.

Scientists realize how difficult it is to discover and develop a new medicine. They know that a result can occur at any time in a program that can require its immediate termination. There are unfortunate cases where a rare side effect is detected after a new medicine has been on the market, resulting in that medicine being discontinued. Clearly, everyone associated with this program was very disappointed. But people quickly moved on to other projects with the potential for meeting other major medical needs.

Patients also expressed their disappointment when the T/A program was halted. Shortly after the public announcement, Jeff Kindler received the following note from Ms. Nancy Loving, Executive Director of Womenheart, the National Coalition for Women with Heart Disease based in Washington, DC:

> On behalf of the 8,000,000 American women living with heart disease, I want to express our heartfelt sorrow and disappointment that you had to make the difficult decision to terminate the torcetrapib trial. So many of us had our hopes riding high on this drug and share what must be your company's very painful sense of loss. But I also want you to know how grateful we are to the Pfizer research scientists, and I appreciate how hard they work to save our lives and improve the quality of our lives. Please convey to them our deepest thanks for all their efforts and encourage them to move forward with even more life-saving discoveries. Our lives are depending on them.

Did the Pfizer scientists feel their work was wasted? While this outcome was disappointing, a number of advances and breakthroughs were made that are having beneficial effects in other programs. For one thing, knowledge was gained in fundamental cholesterol metabolism and cholesterol transport. Second, the spray-dried dispersion (SDD) technology developed for torcetrapib has now been applied to poorly soluble molecules in other programs, thereby demonstrating the broad applicability of SDD technology. In addition, Pfizer scientists were able to determine the three-dimensional structure of CETP using novel X-ray crystallography techniques that can also have application to other programs. Overall, a great deal has been learned. But this was of small consolation on December 1, 2006.

The views of a major critic of the pharmaceutical industry are also interesting to note. Here is an editorial from the *New York Times* of December 5, 2006.

> The discovery that a promising experimental cholesterol drug can be deadly is a financial blow to the manufacturer and a sharp disappointment to doctors and patients who had been hoping for another breakthrough in the fight against heart disease. It is also a sobering reminder that pioneering drug research is a risky business both to patients who take unproven drugs in clinical trials and to companies that bet a good portion of their research budgets on them.

> The drug in this case was torcetrapib, made by Pfizer, the world's largest drug maker. Pfizer had poured almost a billion dollars into developing the drug and had high hopes that it would rejuvenate the company's near-term financial prospects.

> Unlike statins, which fight heart disease by lowering the amount of "bad" cholesterol in the blood, torcetrapib was the front-runner in a new class of drugs that try to raise the level of "good" cholesterol. It was precisely the kind of product we want the industry to focus on; not a "me too" drug that markets a merely incremental advance over some existing therapy but a wholly new approach that could spur a huge leap forward in the battle against heart disease.

As will be depicted again and again in the examples used in this book, the discovery and development of new medicines is a long process that costs hundreds of millions of dollars. Anyone who expounds otherwise is clearly uninformed. The challenging work involved can be frustrating and disappointing. But, when it is successful and results in a new drug that benefits millions of people around the world, it is incredibly fulfilling.

PART *II*

THE ROLE OF PHARMACEUTICAL R&D IN HEALTH CARE

MOST PEOPLE know little or nothing about the research done in the pharmaceutical industry. Too many believe that the essence of drug discovery is carried out in academic labs and that industry simply licenses these drugs, then manufactures and sells them. This prejudice is reinforced by ubiquitous television images of the industry which show pills rolling off an assembly line. Critics of our industry also claim that new medicines add little value. Rather, new drugs are portrayed as glorified versions of older, out-of-patent generics; the new versions simply add increased costs to the health care system but provide little in terms of added benefits. And, if this isn't enough, there are those who believe that real innovation occurs in the biotech industry and that "Big Pharma" doesn't have a clue about how to make real breakthroughs.

The chapters in this section seek to correct these misconceptions. The interdependency between academic labs and industrial labs is discussed in Chapter 4 using as an example a very exciting new approach for treating autoimmune diseases like rheumatoid arthritis and psoriasis. Chapter 5 reviews the value that new medicines bring in actually *reducing* the nation's healthcare bill as demonstrated with a novel agent that helps patients to quit smoking. Anyone who doubts Big Pharma's innovation will be surprised by the last chapter in this section, which describes an entirely new approach to treating AIDS.

CHAPTER 4

DRUGS ARE DISCOVERED BY ACADEMIA

I**T IS** infuriating for a researcher in Pharmaceutical R&D to hear comments such as this:

> Innovative research is done mainly by taxpayer funded research—government and universities funded by the NIH usually in universities and government labs and now in smaller biotech companies.[1]

This quote is not from a commentator unfamiliar with health care. It comes from Dr. Marcia Angell, the former Editor-in-Chief of the *New England Journal of Medicine*. This view is too common. In fact, a survey carried out by Consensus Research in 2003 found that only 27% of the public assign the credit for discovery of new medicines to pharmaceutical companies.[2] And yet, the Pharmaceutical Research and Manufacturers Association found that 90% of new medicines are both discovered and developed by private industry.

Worried that American taxpayers should be sharing more in the profits of the pharmaceutical industry, Congress commissioned a study to determine which of the top-selling drugs had their origins in support by the National Institutes of Health (NIH). This report, prepared by the Department of Health and Human Services (HHS), was issued in July 2001.[3] Key to this report was a thorough investigation by the NIH into the 47 drugs on the market which at that time had sales of $500 million or more. By their own admission, only *four* of the 47 drugs were associated with Federal patent ties. Furthermore, two of these four were the same drug (epoetin). The other 43 drugs were discovered and developed by industry with no federal investment. When it comes to how and by whom drugs are discovered, there is a major disconnect between reality and public perception.

The important role of the NIH in the elucidation of basic science is brilliantly described in another HHS paper, "Report to Congress on Affordability of Inventions and Products," which was issued July 2004.[4]

> The NIH was established with the mission of science in pursuit of fundamental knowledge about the nature and behavior of living systems and the application of that knowledge to extend healthy life and reduce the burdens of illness and disability. In those instances when such research leads to a novel technology, it is the role of the NIH and recipients of NIH funds to disseminate the research findings and, as appropriate,

pursue further development to bring technologies to practical application to benefit the public.

The NIH has a role to play in the early-stage development of technologies that are later brought to market by its licensees or commercial collaborators. The final product, whether it is a therapeutic, a diagnostic, or a medical device, is often the result of a host of discoveries contributed over the years by numerous university, government, or commercial laboratories. The NIH typically contributes to the understanding of basic and clinical biology (such as the pathogenesis of a disease, the immunological or genetic processes associated with a disease, etc.) that helps in guiding translational research toward producing a cure or therapy.

The NIH plays a critical role in funding important biomedical research that provides broad benefits not just to the pharmaceutical industry but to society in general. Furthermore, the fact is that the vast majority of basic biological research is done in academia. But one must distinguish between important theoretical work and the application of this work in discovering and developing new medicines. Basic research is not drug discovery. The following story shows the misconceptions that abound in the respective roles of Industry and Academia. In 2004 a story[5] in *Chemical and Engineering News* described Xalatan, an important medicine used to treat glaucoma, in the following way:

> The drug was developed in the early 1980s at Columbia University and licensed to Pharmacia Corporation, now Pfizer. NIH, through the National Eye Institute, contributed more than $4 million to support the development of this drug.

Even a sophisticated reader would infer that the big, bad pharmaceutical company hoodwinked the unassuming scientists at Columbia and the NIH, thereby extracting hundreds of million of dollars out of the health care system. But, here are some important facts that tell the real story.

The NIH funded research carried out by Professor Laszlo Bito at Columbia University during the late 1970s and early 1980s. Dr. Bito hypothesized that certain molecules (prostaglandins) that are naturally occurring in the body could lower intraocular pressure (IOP). At the time, this was considered a radical idea because larger dose of prostaglandins had been shown to *increase* IOP. Dr. Bito discovered that, in very small doses, prostaglandins could actually *lower* IOP. Since persistent elevated pressure in the eye is a key cause of glaucoma, the potential for using prostaglandins to treat this disease became apparent. With Dr. Bito's important insight, the hard work of drug development process could *begin*. Pharmacia did what Columbia and the NIH could not do: it began looking for specific compounds that mimic the desired chemistry, tested them in animal models, tested them in people for safety and efficacy, provided data to satisfy regulators, and finally—12 years and hundreds of millions of dollars later—introduced an important new product, Xalatan, for the treatment of glaucoma.

It must be pointed out that this type of successful enterprise is more the exception than the rule. Most similar ventures led to huge investments by the pharmaceutical company with zero gain. The element of risk is endured entirely by industry and not the university.

The story of Xalatan is a successful one for Pharmacia (now part of Pfizer), for Columbia, for Dr. Bito, and, most of all, for patients and physicians. Pfizer has a successful product. Columbia earned $31 million dollars from Pfizer in 2003 alone, and it will earn more than $100 million over the life of the Xalatan license for research conducted in its labs paid for with taxpayer funds. Dr. Bito has earned a substantial portion of those royalties. But the big winner is the patient: Xalatan is now the number one prescribed IOP-lowering agent in the United States, and over 100 million prescriptions are written worldwide.

Academic insights are incredibly important in the genesis of the discovery of new medicines. However, these insights are not easily or cheaply translated into effective drugs. A recent paper strongly underscores this point. Zycher, DiMasi, and Milne compiled summary case histories of 35 drug classes to determine the respective contributions of the public and private sectors.[6] They found that private sector research was responsible for central advances in basic science for seven, in applied science for 34, and in the development of drugs yielding improved clinical performance or manufacturing processes for 28. Basically, it is unlikely that any of these drugs would have been available to patients without the major contributions of pharmaceutical companies. The authors go on to say that their study does not dispute the importance of publicly funded research carried out at the NIH, universities and research institutes. However, they point out that "… the scientific contributions of the private sector also have been crucial, but have been weighted heavily toward the applied science of discovering ways to exploit the findings of basic research in pursuit of treatments and cures for adverse medical conditions."

A successful academic–industry interface is crucial in discovering new medicines. The following story, involving the search for a novel drug to treat autoimmune diseases, provides an excellent model for how this works.

THE JAK-3 STORY

Autoimmune diseases are those in which an aberration causes the body to react against itself. The causes of each of these diseases are relatively poorly understood. The diseases themselves are quite varied in nature and include conditions as diverse as psoriasis, Type 1 diabetes, and rheumatoid arthritis. A medicine that could be used to dampen an overactive immune system would be of great value to patients who suffer from such disorders.

In addition, sometimes we want to decrease the activity of the immune system of other patients. Specifically, people who undergo an organ transplantation, such as a kidney or a pancreas, need effective medicines that prevent the body from rejecting the donated organ. A drug that could turn down the immune system could therefore meet a variety of major medical needs.

Back in 1993 Dr. Paul Changelian, a scientist in Pfizer's immune suppression group in Groton, Connecticut, was seeking such a drug. The specific mission of the group at this time was to find an alternative to cyclosporine A (CsA), the medicine of choice for preventing organ rejection. CsA acts by blocking the function of the T-cell, a key component of the immune system. Ironically, one of CsA's main side effects is toxicity to the kidney. Thus, the drug that patients need to prevent their immune system from rejecting their new kidney causes harm to this same kidney. As a result, kidneys last only about 10 years after being transplanted. Given the shortage of kidneys for transplantation, an alternative to CsA, which would prolong the viability of a transplanted kidney, as well as other organs, would have tremendous value. The scientific challenge was to find a new way to achieve this.

As part of his search, in the summer of 1993, Paul decided to attend the "Federation of American Society for Experimental Biology (FASEB) Summer Conference on Lymphocyte and Antibodies" being held in Vermont. He almost didn't attend this meeting because his wife, pregnant with their second son, was not feeling well. Fortunately for medical science, they decided that she would also go to Vermont and Paul was able to attend the meeting.

While at this meeting, Paul ran into an old acquaintance, Dr. John O'Shea, a researcher at the NIH. As scientists are wont to do, Paul and John discussed their current projects. When Paul told John that he was hunting for drug targets that could produce immune suppression, John mentioned that his lab had just discovered a particular enzyme from a class known as kinases that could play a role in immune function.[7] This enzyme is a member of the Janus family of kinases and became more commonly known as JAK-3. JAK-3 was shown to control signaling by the interleukin-2 (IL-2) receptor, a key growth factor for T lymphocytes, the cells responsible for the rejection of a transplanted kidney. Paul was greatly intrigued by these findings, but he did have a concern. At that time, other data suggested that IL-2 was not the only growth factor used by T cells, and blocking it via the JAK-3 pathway might not be sufficient for immune suppression. Once again scientists had arrived at the starting point in their quest for a medical breakthrough. The only road forward was to invent a molecule that blocked JAK-3. Such a discovery was needed to test the hypothesis that modulation of this pathway could help patients with autoimmune disease.

The first thing that Paul and his Pfizer colleagues needed was access to JAK-3. This was achieved by establishing a Material Transfer Agreement (MTA) with the O'Shea lab. Many years ago, MTAs were unheard of. But gone are the days of scientists freely exchanging lab materials with no strings attached. MTAs must now be in place before collaborations occur in order to protect the rights of all involved. In this case, the MTA allowed the Pfizer scientists to prepare the biological materials necessary for building a JAK-3 assay. Having an assay is critical because it allowed Paul and his colleagues to measure if any chemicals could inhibit JAK-3 to even a weak extent. In fact, hundreds of thousands of compounds were tested in the search for such an inhibitor.

However, once the project was underway at Pfizer, it became clear that formal collaboration with the O'Shea lab would benefit both groups. They needed the freedom to discuss their ideas about the biochemistry and cell biology of lymphocytes. To allow this, a Cooperative Research and Development Agreement (CRADA) was established between Pfizer and the NIH for this project.

A bit of history of the CRADA is in order.

With the goals of promoting the timely transfer of technology from government laboratories to the private sector and improving the competitiveness of U.S. industry, Congress passed the Federal Technology Transfer Act (FTTA) of 1986. The FTTA allows a federal government laboratory (NCI, NIH, the Veterans Administration, etc.) to enter into CRADAs with private entities, including the pharmaceutical industry. The nongovernment party to a CRADA is termed a "Collaborator." With a CRADA, federal agencies can conduct collaborative research with such Collaborators and protect intellectual property that may be developed, while allowing government resources to be applied to interests in the private sector. A CRADA is not a procurement contract for goods or services, nor is it a grant agreement. The government party in a CRADA may provide personnel, facilities, equipment, and expertise to perform the collaborative research. The Collaborator may provide personnel, facilities, equipment, expertise, and funding. A CRADA is the only contracting mechanism under which a federal agency can receive direct funding from industry.

Since any research-oriented federal agency can enter into CRADAs, there is significant variation in the terms of these agreements, with each agency tailoring the CRADA somewhat to meet its specific situation. In addition, CRADAs can differ as to scope, with some being limited to specific studies or areas of research and development and others covering the entire development of a product. However, features common to most CRADAs include (1) shared ownership of data generated under the CRADA, (2) government ownership of intellectual property developed by government employees, with the Collaborator receiving an option to negotiate for a license, (3) an automatic nonexclusive royalty-free license to the government to any intellectual property developed under the CRADA, including intellectual property exclusively licensed to Collaborator or developed solely by Collaborator, (4) limited Collaborator rights to terminate the CRADA early, and (5) a government right to require the Collaborator, under extraordinary circumstances, to grant licenses to third parties to Collaborator-owned or exclusively licensed intellectual property developed under the CRADA.

Despite several nonstandard risks and burdens to the Collaborator, CRADAs can create a win–win situation for the federal agency and industry. In return for granting access to basic science or other government resources to the Collaborator, the applied research can be broadly disseminated to the benefit of the public, which is in keeping with the mission of the research-oriented federal partner. It is important to note that the work done under the CRADA between Pfizer and the NIH for this program resulted in several joint publications from the Pfizer and NIH labs.[8a,b] This is an excellent example of the respective roles played by academia and industry in the discovery of new medicines. A fundamental observation was made by John O'Shea and his colleagues. Paul Changelian and the Pfizer team translated this observation to discover a potential new medicine.

As was stated earlier, when this program began in 1993, it was unclear whether a JAK-3 inhibitor alone would be sufficient for immune suppression. However, confidence in this target grew about a year later thanks to a remarkable series of papers that emerged from the NIH and the University of Tokyo.[9a,b] These researchers found that cell signaling through the JAK-3 pathway was required not just for one cytokine receptor, IL-2, but also for five other cytokine receptors as well: IL-4, IL-7, IL-9, IL-15, and IL-21. Furthermore, it was predicted that patients with defects in JAK-3 would be severely immunocompromised. This was demonstrated in 1995 when it was found that a patient with severe combined immunodeficiency disease ("Bubble Boy Syndrome") had a genetic defect that prevented the production of JAK-3.[10] It was clear then that JAK-3 was an exciting target. The race was now on to discovery a JAK-3 inhibitor for clinical testing.

Once the enzyme was in hand and cell assays were built, the Pfizer chemical library was screened in search of molecules that could inhibit JAK-3. By the end of 1995, an initial lead molecule was identified. This compound, code named CP-352,664, demonstrated weak but reproducible inhibition against JAK-3. Over the next 5 years, Pfizer scientists synthesized and screened about 3000 compounds analyzing each for potency, selectivity for JAK-3, and activity in a mouse heart transplant model. These studies resulted in the identification of the first JAK-3 inhibitor to enter preclinical development, CP-690,550, in August 2000, 7 years after Changelian's trip to Vermont.

At this point, one can usually begin planning for clinical studies. Unlike many other therapeutic areas, however, more than just rodent or small animal data were needed to convince clinicians to try this new transplant drug. Kidney transplant patients wait several years to get an appropriate kidney. Furthermore, even though the current drugs are not without problems, the surgeons can virtually guarantee that their new kidney will survive another 5–10 years with current therapy. Thus, in order for us to convince transplant physicians to take a chance on CP-690,550, the drug needed to work in a rigorous model of kidney transplantation in a more closely related species. Studies in monkeys were carried out by Dr. Dominic Borie and his team at Stanford University. This is another example of the need for industry–university collaborations. This group, one of the best in the world, had performed studies with a number of transplantation drugs that were already on the market. While interested in CP-690,550, they cautioned the Pfizer team not to expect too much from this first foray into the immune suppression arena.

Much to their surprise, the actual results proved extraordinarily positive. CP-690,550-treated monkeys had transplanted kidneys that showed no evidence of tox-icity or tissue death. These results were much better than those seen with animals treated with either placebo or CsA. The CP-690,550-treated kidneys looked so healthy that one of the researchers questioned whether the biopsy sample was truly from a transplanted kidney. Pictures of these kidneys are shown in Figure 4.1. CP-690,550 proved to be the most potent and safe compound that the Stanford group had ever tested.[11] It was now time to test this compound in humans.

In order to get a rapid read-out of whether the potent CP-690,550 immunosup-pressive properties would translate to humans, in 2002 Pfizer sponsored a study with key medical advisors to test this compound in patients with severe psoriasis, a disease caused by a dysfunctional immune system. Again, excellent results were seen. People treated with 30 mg of CP-690,550 twice a day for 2 weeks showed remarkable improvement as illustrated in Figure 4.2. Without a doubt, CP-690,550 has excellent immunosuppressive properties in this patient population.

Renal Allograft Biopsy

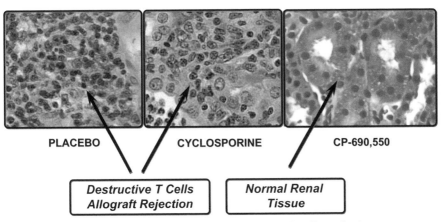

PLACEBO   CYCLOSPORINE   CP-690,550

Destructive T Cells
Allograft Rejection

Normal Renal
Tissue

Figure 4.1   CP-690,550 in monkey transplant rejection studies. See color insert.

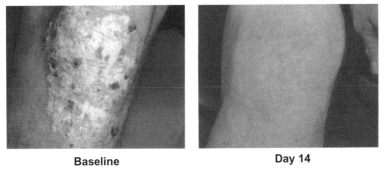

Baseline   **Day 14**

Figure 4.2   Phase 1 study of CP-690,550 given twice daily at a dose of 30 mg in volunteers with psoriasis.

With these results in hand, studies with CP-690,550 in preventing kidney rejection and rheumatoid arthritis began in early 2005. Rheumatoid arthritis (RA) is a particularly debilitating progressive disease. At its worst, it can cause deformities of the hands, feet, knees, and other joints, making simple daily tasks such as getting dressed or driving a car very difficult. There is no cure. People with RA will take various medications such as nonsteroidal anti-inflammatory drugs (NSAIDs) or cyclooxygenase-2 inhibitors (COX-2s) to relieve their pain. They also can be prescribed disease-modifying antirheumatic drugs (DMARDs) such as methotrexate, which slow disease progression. However, the predominant agents now used are "biologics," the products of novel technologies. These are highly targeted medications that block mediators of inflammation such as tumor necrosis factor (TNF) or cytokines like IL-1. Unfortunately, these drugs are proteins or protein-like and

◆ **Protocol Design for CP-690,550 RA Study**
  • **Randomized, Double-blind, Placebo Controlled, Multi-center Study**
  • **6-Weeks of Dosing in 262 Patients Who Failed anti-TNF Biological or Methotrexate**
◆ **Primary Endpoint: % Responders (ACR 20 Response*) at 6 Weeks**

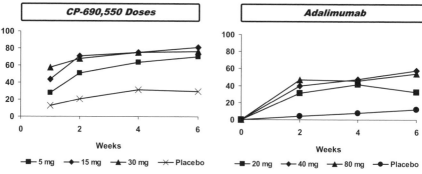

Figure 4.3   Rheumatoid arthritis study.

cannot be taken orally. They must be administered by either injection or intravenous infusion, are difficult to store, and are very costly to produce.

As described earlier, by inhibiting JAK-3, CP-690,550 can inhibit the production of multiple cytokines, which are mediators of inflammation. Furthermore, it can be administered daily as a pill. Theoretically, this JAK-3 inhibitor could be highly effective in RA. To test this hypothesis, a Phase 2 study was carried out to determine the efficacy of CP-690,550 in RA in 262 patients. A high hurdle was set for this study in that it included only RA patients who had already failed improvement when treated with either the DMARD methotrexate or a biological inhibitor of TNF, adalimumab.

The results for CP-690,550 in relieving the signs and symptoms of RA were stunning. Not only was CP-690,550 effective in these patents, but the level of efficacy was greater than that normally seen in RA patients who can get relief with the biological TNF inhibitor. These results are depicted in Figure 4.3. (It should be noted that these graphs do not represent a head-to-head comparison, but rather the adalimumab results are included for reference.)

These results with CP-690,550 in RA, if confirmed by ongoing Phase 3 studies, could change the paradigm in treating this crippling disease. CP-690,550 could prove to be more efficacious than current treatments and is simply administered. More work still needs to be done with CP-690,550, and late-stage clinical studies in both RA and the prevention of kidney transplant rejection continue. But CP-690,550 could prove to be an extremely exciting new therapy for patients suffering from autoimmune diseases. Paul Changelian captures the current status very well:

The story began when my second son was in utero. He is now a 14-year-old eighth grader. If everything goes well, by the time he goes to his junior prom, 17 years after

I went to the scientific meeting in the woods of Vermont, CP-690,550 might make it to the pharmacy shelves and to the patients who need it.

Or it might not. It is a tough game—but always worth playing.

This 14-year journey began with two scientists, one from the NIH and one from Pfizer, attending a conference in Vermont and talking about their respective work. Drugs are not discovered in academia. But the basic science done in this realm often provides an important starting point for subsequent medical breakthroughs.

CHAPTER 5

NEW MEDICINES ADD COSTS BUT LITTLE BENEFIT

THERE IS a view that Americans are "over-medicated" and that this reliance on pills is driving the rise in health costs in the United States. This is incorrect. As shown in Figure 5.1, the percentage of spending on pharmaceuticals in the United States has remained relatively constant for the last 50 years and amounts to about 10% of overall health care costs. This statistic surprises many patients. Their confusion is a result of the fact that, unlike the costs for hospital or physician care, the costs of medicines are borne at least in part by patients, and price increases or changes in insurance plan payments are passed on directly to the consumer. These are seen as increases in out-of-pocket expenses passed on by insurers as "co-pays."

As patients' expenses for medicines have increased, people have begun to question their value. Even more concerning has been the tendency for health providers to limit the access to new medicines by minimizing reimbursement. This view that reducing access to medicines in order to reduce overall health care costs is short-sighted. The proper use of drugs can limit costly hospitalizations, which drive up health care costs. This can be fostered by providing access to medicines along with the necessary support to encourage healthy habits such as improved diet and exercise. These actions just don't improve clinical outcomes but allow people to work more productively.

There are many studies which show that the proper use of medicines can often result in *savings* to the overall health care system. For illustrative purposes, three will be described. The first case involves the care of people with schizophrenia, a disease that carries economic, clinical, and personal burdens. In the early 1990s in an attempt to rein in health care costs, the State of New Hampshire decided to limit Medicaid drug-reimbursement benefits on the use of psychotropic agents by schizophrenic patients. Presumably the rationale for this was that these noninstitutionalized patients had moderate schizophrenia that could be controlled with minimal medication. The "cap" for these patients was set at three prescriptions per month. Soumerai and colleagues studied the impact of this cap on acute mental health service usage. They hypothesized that reducing access to these drugs would increase not just emergency mental health services but also hospitalizations.

As they published in the *New England Journal of Medicine*,[1] the Soumerai team showed that the cap had an immediate impact in reducing the use of

---

Drug Truths: Dispelling the Myths About Pharma R&D, by John L. LaMattina
Copyright © 2009 John Wiley & Sons, Inc.

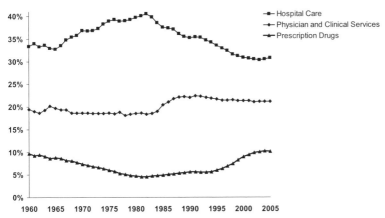

Figure 5.1   Share of national health care spent in each category, 1960–2005. (Source: CMS, available at: http://www.cms.gov.)

antipsychotic drugs, lithium, and other medications in the range of 15–49%. Over the course of a year, this resulted in a per-patient savings of $57. Unfortunately, these savings were counterbalanced by a coincident increase of one to two visits per patient per month to community health centers and sharp increases in the use of emergency mental health services and partial hospitalizations. This resulted in an average increase in mental health care costs of $1530 per patient while the cap was in place. Needless to say, the cap was discontinued and the use of medications and mental health services reverted to baseline levels.

The conclusion of these authors was quite telling:

> Limits on coverage for the costs of prescription drugs can increase the use of acute mental health services among low-income patients with chronic mental illnesses and increase costs to the government, even aside from the increases caused in pain and suffering on the part of the patients.

Clearly, limiting access to these medicines was harmful to patients and ineffective in saving money.

The second example shows the benefits of *increasing* access to medicines, particularly in the overall management of a chronic disease like diabetes. This was demonstrated in the landmark Asheville Project. In an effort to improve the health of their citizenry, Asheville, North Carolina created a program granting diabetics free access to both prescription drugs and overall services if patients enrolled in a care-management program. By providing complete care for these patients, Asheville hoped to drive down overall costs while improving the health of these individuals. Cranor et al.[2] reported on the progress made with this project after 5 years.

At the start of the study, overall per patient annual cost of health care was on average $7082, with $1153 of this attributed to the cost of medicines. Over the 5-year period, with free access to the needed medications, Asheville's drug bill for each diabetic rose to $3095. However, the total annual patient cost dropped to $4661.

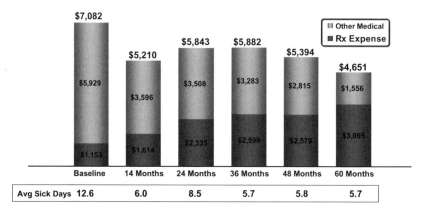

CPSM 5.3.0

Figure 5.2   Asheville Project.

Furthermore, Asheville didn't have to wait 5 years for the benefits to be seen. As shown in Figure 5.2, significant savings were realized after 14 months.

It is clear that this program paid significant dividends. Not only have medical expenses dropped by more than one-third, but the overall health of these patients improved as measured by a greater than 50% drop in sick days. The authors estimated that this increase in worker productivity was worth $18,000 for one employer group annually. And yet this occurred despite the near tripling of the costs of the prescription medicines used. It is well established that vigorous control of diabetes through diet, exercise, and, yes, drugs can provide improved long-term outcomes and reduce the dreaded complications of diabetes such as blindness, kidney failure, and heart disease. The leaders of Asheville deserve a great deal of credit for having the foresight to undertake this program. It provides another example of the value of medicines.

The last example comes in the treatment of AIDS. In the late 1990s, highly active antiretroviral therapy (HAART, also known as "triple therapy") was introduced. The impact of HAART on the survival of AIDS patients was stunning as shown in Figure 5.3a. However, triple therapy was viewed to be expensive, and so questions arose as to increased costs of care for patients with HIV. Bozzette et al.[3] therefore studied 2864 patients representative of American adults receiving care for HIV infection beginning in January 1996. At that point, total monthly care was approximately $1800. As one would have predicted, 18 months later the drug bill for HAART resulted in a 34% increase in drug costs for these patients. However, the overall health care expense was down to $1521 per month, a 41% decrease (Figure 5.3b). Obviously, HAART was affording AIDS patients overall better health. More importantly, they were living longer and contributing their skills and energy to society, family, and friends.

These examples all show that new medicines not only improve the quality of life for millions of patients but also reduce overall costs to the health care system. As health care providers around the globe search for ways to improve health and

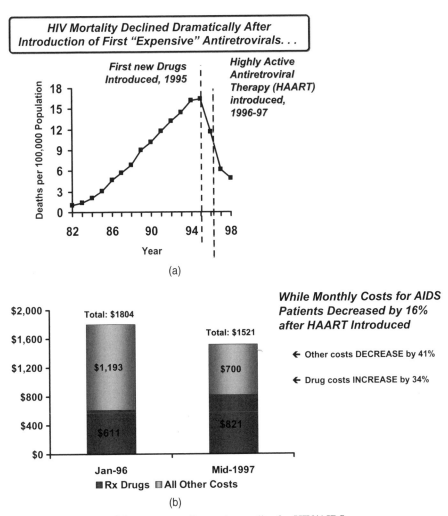

Figure 5.3   Impact of drugs on spending and mortality for HIV/AIDS.

reduce costs, there is an obvious place where inroads can be made, namely, smoking cessation. Smoking is quite simply the leading preventable cause of mortality. Tobacco causes fatal and disabling diseases including lung cancer, heart disease, stroke, and respiratory diseases. In addition, nonsmokers, who are exposed to second-hand smoke, have higher rates of illnesses than those who breathe clean air. Children are especially vulnerable as parental smoking contributes to increased rates of asthma, bronchitis, colds, and pneumonia.

There are estimated to be 1.3 billion smokers worldwide. It is believed that 1.6 million deaths in the United States and Europe occur every year as a result of smoking leading to $150 billion per year in costs due to smoking-related illnesses. The medical need for a reliable and safe treatment to help smokers quit is urgent and obvious.

THE DISCOVERY AND DEVELOPMENT OF CHANTIX

The origin of smoking in the Western world can be traced back to the early days of American colonization. Thomas Hariot, in his "A Brief and True Report of the New Found Land of Virginia 1588," provided the following description:

> Natives smoke "an herb called uppowoc … the fumes purge superfluous phlegm and gross humors from the body by opening all the pores and passages. Thus its use not only preserves the body, but if there are any obstructions it breaks them up. By this means the natives keep in excellent health, without many of the grievous diseases which often afflict us in England.

However, at the beginning of the seventeenth century, King James I issued a scathing attack on this habit imported from the Colonies.[4]

> Smoking is a custom loathsome to the eye, hateful to the nose, harmful to the brain, dangerous to the lungs, and in the black, stinking fume thereof nearest resembling the horrible Stygian smoke of the pit that is bottomless.

Given that smoking was viewed as such a vile practice more than 400 years ago, how has it become so popular? Unbeknownst to the settlers of the New World, smoking tobacco resulted in brain exposure to nicotine, one of the most addictive substances known. Nicotine binds to the $\alpha4\beta2$ receptor in the central nervous system (CNS). Once nicotine binds in the CNS, it results in the release of another substance called dopamine, which, in turn, is linked to reward. Smokers become dependent on these modest yet pleasurable emissions of dopamine. When a smoker tries to quit, the craving and withdrawal symptoms experienced are due to slumping levels of dopamine.

In 1993 Drs. Jim Heym and David Schulz at Pfizer's laboratories in Groton, Connecticut, began a program seeking partial agonists of the nicotine binding site, the $\alpha4\beta2$ cholinergic receptor. Their rationale in seeking such a compound was straightforward. By having a partial agonist—a compound that would bind to the receptor as nicotine does but which didn't fully activate this receptor—one could have a drug that had the potential to relieve craving and withdrawal when quitting but would also block the reinforcing effects if one did try to smoke a cigarette.

Back in 1993, all of this was theoretical. The team really needed to identify compounds that were partial agonists of the $\alpha4\beta2$ receptor to test these hypotheses. For a number of years, dozens of Pfizer scientists worked to measure the binding of compounds to both rat and human nicotine receptors, to determine neurochemical potency and efficacy, and to measure toleration and oral bioavailability of test compounds.

The key insight that enabled the program to flourish was made by a chemist, Dr. Jotham Coe. Jotham had once been a smoker but was fortunate enough to quit in his thirties. His father was a lifelong smoker who died of emphysema, so Jotham knew first-hand of the pain caused by this addiction. Jotham and his chemistry colleagues started with an alkaloid found in plants, cytosine, which was known to have modest binding potential to nicotine receptors. In studying cytosine's structure, he s-(-)-Nicotine   Varenicline

Figure 5.4   The structures of nicotine and varenicline.

recognized that it contained elements similar to morphine, a molecule Jotham had worked on earlier in his career. This observation led him to produce a series of compounds with potent α4β2 binding activity, and this work has been summarized in recent publications.[5,6] These efforts ultimately produced varenicline, a partial agonist of the α4β2 receptor. For a chemist, the structure of varenicline is deceptively simple as shown in Figure 5.4. Varenicline was first tested in human volunteers in 1999.

Normally, smokers are excluded from early clinical trials because nicotine dependency complicates factors when evaluating the safety and toleration of an experimental medicine. However, since varenicline was designed to be used in smokers, they were included in the earliest studies. These volunteers were not recruited so that they could be helped to quit. The intent was simply to measure safety and toleration in the type of patients the drug would be used to treat. The volunteers in the multiple-dose Phase 1 study smoked an average of 20–25 cigarettes per day. They were treated either with placebo or with varenicline (1 mg, twice a day) for 14 days. Those in the placebo group showed no difference in cigarette consumption during these two weeks. However, those on varenicline, despite the fact that they hadn't intended to quit smoking, smoked only 5–6 cigarettes per day. This was a very encouraging result.

In every successful drug program, there is usually an "aha" moment when a certain result becomes available and indicates that a new medicine may actually emerge from the program. For the nicotine partial agonist project, this occurred when the results of a major Phase 2 study were revealed. This study *was* intended to show if varenicline could help smokers quit. Three doses of varenicline were compared to placebo and to a marketed smoking cessation treatment, bupropion (an antidepressant agent sold as Zyban for smoking cessation). Figure 5.5 depicts what was found. Varenicline clearly worked and, at 1 mg twice a day, it was significantly more efficacious than the marketed agent. Furthermore, varenicline was well-tolerated, with the most common side effect being nausea. For those who took 1 mg of varenicline twice a day for 6 weeks, almost half had kicked the habit for at least 4 weeks with no major side effects. Although a major Phase 3 program was still needed to generate the data required for regulatory approval, the team was very excited. Varenicline had the potential to be a major medical breakthrough.

At this point, the Development team met with the FDA to find out what they required from a large Phase 3 program. Meetings of this type are critical. The FDA has strong views about what information should be generated in a particular Phase 3 program in order to satisfy their demands that a new drug is safe and efficacious. In this case, the FDA was most interested in the long-term, not 4-week, quit rates

% of Smokers Who Quit For 4 Weeks

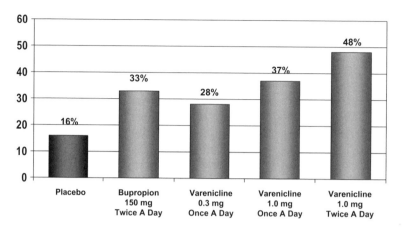

Each group has 125 patients who were dosed continuously for 6 weeks

Figure 5.5   Phase II study.

resulting from varenicline therapy. The Phase 3 program, which was carried out at medical centers around the world, tested placebo, bupropion, and two doses of varenicline: 0.5 mg (twice a day) and 1 mg (twice a day). Patients on varenicline were dosed for 12 weeks and were then followed for a year. After 12 weeks of varenicline therapy, roughly 44% of the patients on drug had quit smoking. A year later, half of these stayed cigarette-free.

These results, along with massive amounts of other data, were filed with the FDA in November 2005. Recognizing the importance of a drug to treat nicotine addiction, the FDA gave varenicline a Priority Review Status and within 6 months approved the drug, sold as Chantix, as an aid to smoking cessation on May 11, 2006. Similarly, approval was granted in Europe by the European Medicines Agency (EMEA), where the drug is sold as Champix.

Besides having a medicine to help them quit, smokers also need to have help in motivating themselves to stop. Therefore, Chantix users also have access at no cost to the GETQUIT™ support plan, a multichannel approach customized to each patient to help provide support to overcome their nicotine addiction. This program is designed to ensure success by encouraging compliance and to provide support for the patient to remain smoke-free.

The R&D Team has received international recognition for their efforts in bringing Chantix to patients. They received the "Scrip Award for the Best Small Molecule Drug" for 2006. They also received the "Prix Galien Prize" in 2007 for the Best Pharmaceutical Agent. While this recognition is well-deserved, the team's most rewarding moments come from patients who have benefited from Chantix. These testimonials are received daily, but the following one comes from a Pfizer colleague and so it hits a bit closer to home.

My mother has been a life-long smoker—she's 73 now. About 3 years ago she had to have surgery to repair an aortic abdominal aneurysm. The number one cause of "Triple A's" is smoking. While this should have been a strong motivator to quit, she couldn't do it.

Then, about a year and a half ago, she started having pains in her legs. She was diagnosed with peripheral artery disease. Again, smoking is one of the top causes for that. Over the last year, she has had seven vascular surgeries on her legs to improve her circulation. Her surgeon told her before the first surgery she must quit smoking because there is a high incidence of graft failure that's inherent in the kind of graft surgery she had, even for non-smokers.

She tried. She couldn't quit. Her grafts failed.

By surgery number six, her surgeon told her that if they couldn't get a graft to work in her worst leg, she might have to have an amputation. Luckily, by that time Chantix was on the market. She started Chantix earlier this year and was cigarette-free from the second week she started. She had her most recent graft surgery in May, and I'm happy to say it seems to have taken well. My mom absolutely credits Pfizer and Chantix with her ability to stay off cigarettes.

If Chantix could help someone who smoked for 60 years like my mom, I don't think of it as a therapy—for my family, it's a miracle.

Ordinarily, this would have been the end of the Chantix story. By late 2007, roughly five million smokers around the world had taken Chantix. Translating the results from the clinical trials over two million people would have stopped smoking thanks to their 12 weeks of Chantix therapy. However, routine post-marketing safety reports revealed that a small number of patients showed signs of neuropsychiatric symptoms including changes in behavior, agitation, depressed mood, suicidal ideation, and suicidal behavior. On February 1, 2008 the FDA, after reviewing these reports, identified 491 reports of suicidal thoughts or behaviors possibly linked to Chantix worldwide. As a result of this information, the labeling for Chantix was changed to heighten the awareness of this and to ensure that patients and doctors closely monitor patients during Chantix treatment.[7]

A more thorough discussion of the risk–benefit balance of drug therapy will appear in Chapter 8. But there are some important points to note for this situation. First, in the Chantix controlled Phase 3 trial program, there was no clinically meaningful difference in neuropsychiatric symptoms between patients dosed on placebo as compared to those dosed with Chantix. Oftentimes, the side effects of drugs are not seen until millions of patients have been treated with a new medicine. Second, no data exist for neuropsychiatric symptoms that occur for those patients who quit smoking either "cold turkey" or by other means. Nicotine withdrawal from decades of smoking inevitably would be expected to have some impact on a person's neuropsychiatric state. Third, this anecdote demonstrates how the safety of a medicine is monitored all through its life.

Clearly, health care professionals should monitor patients taking Chantix for behavior and mood changes. But this should not diminish the importance of this medication in getting millions of smokers to quit. The risk–benefit equation for this drug highly favors the benefit side.

Given the importance of reining in health care costs and given the long-term downstream costs caused by nicotine addiction, one would think that, after being approved 2 years ago, Chantix would be universally available from health care providers. That surprisingly is not yet the case. A recent story in *The Daily Telegraph*, an Australian newspaper, revealed that smokers will have to pay for this drug out of their own pockets, despite the fact that it was approved for a government subsidy. Why? Because the Australian Cabinet must approve its ultimate use since the subsidy would cost the Australian government more than $10 million (Australian) per year.[8] Australia is not alone. In early 2008 in the United States, only 30% of patients had coverage for Medicare or Veterans Administration reimbursement.

Some decision makers believe that smoking is a lifestyle choice and so patients should pay for smoking cessation agents. This is short-sighted. The subsequent high costs of lung cancer, heart disease, and so on, will weigh heavily on those health management organizations that do not take advantage of the opportunity to stop smoking as soon as possible. As with the examples given earlier in this chapter, Chantix is another drug that when properly used will result in overall savings to the health care system.

CHAPTER 6

BIG PHARMA HAS FAILED AND SHOULD LEARN FROM BIOTECH SUCCESS

MOST PEOPLE have a soft spot in their heart for the underdog. Children are taught the story of David and Goliath. The legendary Battle of Thermopylae, in which a few hundred Spartan soldiers withstood the massive Persian armies, is a highlight of any treatise on the history of Western Civilization. And the gold medal winning efforts of the collegians who comprised the U.S. hockey team at the 1980 Winter Olympics inspired a nation. Stories of people facing difficult challenges and then overcoming them with hard work, ingenuity, and courage can be inspirational.

The biotech industry is perceived as the "little guy" in the overall scheme of delivering new medicines. Biotech companies are small and lack resources but are portrayed as quick and agile. They are thought of as decisive, not bureaucratic; and scientifically smart, not stuck-in-the mud. The major pharmaceutical companies are contrasted as slow, dumb Goliaths. It is common to read a commentary on R&D productivity in which "Big Pharma" is urged to focus on the manufacture and marketing of new medicines and let small biotech companies do innovative research. Hopefully, the examples in this book demonstrate the value and creativity contributed by a major pharmaceutical company.

Smaller biotech firms do, in fact, play an important role in the search for new medicines. Start-up companies provide a venue for the exploration of more speculative ideas. The first biotech companies had their roots in bioengineering techniques designed to discover large molecules or proteins to treat diseases—work that was largely outside the scope of what was being done in most pharmaceutical companies. They then moved into other forms of protein-based therapies such as antibodies. Now small biotech companies can be founded on a whole gamut of new ideas from the exploration of new technology platforms to the search of a small molecule inhibitor of a newly discovered target to treat diabetes.

A mutual dependency has grown between biotech and Big Pharma. This really is no surprise. A large company like Pfizer has historically had about one-third of its revenues derived from products licensed from other inventors. No matter how much money a company invests in R&D, this is just a small percentage of the funds invested in R&D globally. It is arrogant to believe that any one company has a

Drug Truths: Dispelling the Myths About Pharma R&D, by John L. LaMattina
Copyright © 2009 John Wiley & Sons, Inc.

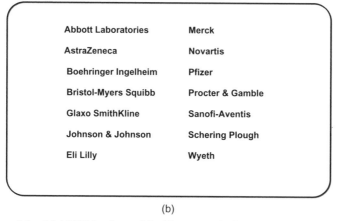

Abbott Laboratories	G.D. Searle	Procter & Gamble
American Cyanamid	Glaxo	Rhone Poulenc
A.H. Robins	Hoechst	Rorer
Astra	Hoffmann-LaRoche	R.P. Scherer
BASF	ICI	Roussel
Beecham Laboratories	Johnson & Johnson	Sandoz
Boehringer Ingelheim	Knoll	Schering Plough
Boots Pharmaceuticals	Eli Lilly	SmithKline
Bristol-Myers	Marion Laboratories	Squibb
Carter-Wallace	Merck	Sterling Drug
Ciba Geigy	Merrell Dow	Upjohn Company
Connaught Laboratories	Monsanto	Warner-Lambert
DuPont Pharmaceuticals	Pfizer	Wellcome
Fisons Corporations	Pharmacia	Zeneca

(a)

Abbott Laboratories	Merck
AstraZeneca	Novartis
Boehringer Ingelheim	Pfizer
Bristol-Myers Squibb	Procter & Gamble
Glaxo SmithKline	Sanofi-Aventis
Johnson & Johnson	Schering Plough
Eli Lilly	Wyeth

(b)

Figure 6.1 (**a**) 1988 Members of the Pharmaceutical Research and Manufacturers Association of America (PhRMA). (**b**) PhRMA members that remain from 1988.

monopoly on the best ideas. In addition, it would also be folly to believe that every project that is run will be successful. Thus, licensing compounds from third parties can serve to fill strategic holes in a company's pipeline or expand a company's capabilities into new areas.

In the 1970s and 1980s, the sources of licensing opportunities for Big Pharma were generally small pharmaceutical companies located around the world that did not have the capabilities or the global presence to reach patients across the world. However, this model began to shift in the 1990s with the consolidation of the pharmaceutical industry. As shown in Figure 6.1a, in 1988 there were over 40 members of the Pharmaceutical Research and Manufacturers Association (PhRMA). After mergers and acquisitions, this number has shrunk considerably (Figure 6.1b). It should be noted that other companies such as Astellas and Amgen have joined PhRMA in recent years and so PhRMA's roster is more than these 14. Industry consolidation has occurred in both Europe and Japan, thus further downsizing the pool of potential licensees from the traditional pharmaceutical industry.

The growing biotech industry has moved into this void. A small company, infused with funds from investors and venture capitalists, can generally take programs only so far—and that is if they are successful. As was described in Chapter 3, as a compound proceeds through clinical development, the program costs increase dramatically. It is not unusual for small companies to seek a Big Pharma partner to assume the costs of the clinical program and the *risk*. A clinical program can kill a small company if the outcome proves to be negative. Alternatively, if the main focus of the biotech company is a single program as can be the case, the Big Pharma partner might simply buy the company outright. In either case, despite the consolidation of the pharmaceutical industry, the in-sourcing of a significant portion of Big Pharma's revenue is likely to continue well into the future and the biotech industry will be an important source of such licensing.

The biotech industry also plays another major role in the delivery of new drugs. There are many diseases that are rare or that occur in relatively small patient populations. As was stated earlier, the R&D costs for the early stages of drug project tend to be similar whether one is seeking treatment for a rare disease or a major one. In order to support its large infrastructure, a Big Pharma company will tend to go after drugs to treat major diseases. A product with peak sales of $100 million is not something that can sustain a major pharmaceutical company. However, such a product can be a major success for a small biotech company. Thus, this industry contributes to finding new medical solutions that are normally eschewed by Big Pharma.

Given that the biotech industry has existed for about 30 years, has it demonstrated superior productivity and business success? This topic is the subject of an excellent book entitled *Science Business* by Professor Gary Pisano of Harvard Business School.[1] In his chapter entitled "The Performance of the Biotech Industry," Pisano rigorously analyzed the history of biotech to date. In looking at R&D productivity, he studied the cumulative spending per new drug produced by each sector from 1985 to 2004. The data showed there was *no difference* in the cost for bringing a compound to market, be it from a biotech firm or Big Pharma. On the theory that biotech's promise is yet to be realized, Pisano questioned this due to the increased R&D spending occurring in biotech along with higher compound attrition rates. He next considered revenue-adjusted productivity with the view that, since drugs vary in their economic impact, this would be a viable productivity assessment. This analysis showed that revenue-adjusted productivity actually greatly favored Big Pharma. A skeptic of Big Pharma might argue that biotech does the creative, more innovative work and that Big Pharma only follows up with "me-too" drugs and so Pisano studied this as well. Again, the data showed little difference in drug novelty between the two sectors. Pisano's conclusions will certainly startle, if not shock, most people:

> The data, despite their limits, would lead us to seriously question the hypothesis that, when it comes to R&D, biotechnology firms are significantly more productive than their large pharmaceutical counterparts. If there is a productivity problem in the

industry, it seems to be equally shared by both big pharmaceutical firms and biotech firms.

Dr. Pisano's conclusion really shouldn't be at all surprising. The challenges that need to be overcome in bringing a new medicine to market are the same regardless of the sector where R&D is done. Selecting a winning target, finding a compound to modulate that target, showing that the compound is safe and effective in people, and demonstrating the economic value that the new medicine brings all are universally difficult. There are no shortcuts. Success rests largely on having talented scientists with creative ideas and a strong motivation to succeed. Neither biotech nor Big Pharma has a monopoly in this.

Innovative solutions are needed not only to come up with treatments for diseases (such as Alzheimer's) for which there are no cures, but also for diseases for which current therapies are suboptimal or perhaps even beginning to fail. The following story describes the discovery of a new medicine that provides new hope for AIDS patients in need of new treatments. It is a project that the uninitiated might have assumed would have been the province of biotech. In fact, it was solved by Big Pharma.

A NEW HYPOTHESIS FOR TREATING AIDS

The development of medicines to control AIDS is one of the great success stories in modern medicine. As a disease, AIDS was first recognized in the early 1980s. In the early days, a person diagnosed with AIDS was essentially being given a death sentence because there were no treatments known. However, through the work of the NIH, regulatory agencies, pharmaceutical companies, and dedicated scientists from around the globe, medicines became available that reduced mortality from AIDS. The fact that these medicines were available to patients in such a relatively short period of time was remarkable. As was described in Chapter 5, with the introduction of Highly Active Antiretroviral Therapy (HAART) by 1996, death rates from AIDS in the United States fell by 70% and HIV transmission to newborns by their HIV-infected mothers was reduced from 25% to 2%. In the Western world, AIDS has been converted from a lethal disease to a chronic disorder managed through a cocktail of drug interventions.[2]

Unfortunately, the virus is developing resistance to current AIDS treatments. People who have had their disease under control for the past 10–15 years are beginning to see their HIV levels slowly rising. There is clearly a need to develop a new generation of medicines to take the place of older treatments in order to keep this disease in check.

Aware of this potential for resistance to existing medicines, scientists have been seeking new approaches to neutralize HIV. One such approach was uncovered in 1996.[3] A small percentage of the population is naturally resistant to AIDS despite having been exposed to HIV. These resistant individuals lack a protein that normally exists on the surface of white blood cells. This deficiency is the result of a deletion

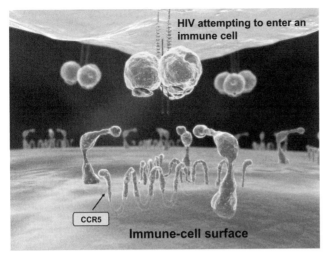

Figure 6.2   HIV Cell Entry *via* the CCR-5 Receptor. See color insert.

in the CCR-5 gene called CCR5-Δ32. This deletion results in a nonfunctional CCR-5 protein. People with two copies of the CCR5-Δ32 gene are resistant to HIV infection. People with one copy of the CCR5-Δ32 gene can be infected with HIV, but disease progression is much slower than what occurs in people with normal CCR-5 function.

What is so special about CCR-5 protein? This protein is a key entry point for HIV to infect a cell (Figure 6.2). If HIV cannot enter a cell, it cannot co-opt the cell's inner workings to reproduce itself. HAART therapy focuses on destroying the virus once it has penetrated a cell. Preventing virus infiltration would provide a novel and complementary approach to treating AIDS.

When the prevalence of this natural immunity to AIDS was studied by geographic region, an interesting trend emerged. The CCR5-Δ32 mutation is not found in the people of sub-Saharan Africa, Asia, or native Americans. Furthermore, the percentage of people with this mutation is relatively low in countries bordering the Mediterranean Sea. However, AIDS immunity occurs in European populations with the highest prevalence of 10–15% seen in Scandinavians. It is believed that this immunity can be traced to bubonic plague ("Black Death") because the causative agent of the plague, *Yersinia pestis*, also utilizes CCR5-Δ32. From 1346 to 1352, bubonic plague killed an estimated 25–40% of Europeans. There were intermittent epidemics after this, the largest being in 1665–1666 ("Great Plague") that killed 15–20% of Europe's population. Many of the survivors were those who lacked CCR5-Δ32.[4,5] Essentially, these plagues hundreds of years ago put selective pressure on Europeans and generated a degree of immunity to the AIDS pandemic. Roughly 2% of the overall population has this genetic mutation that confers AIDS immunity.

These insights into a mode of HIV infection of white blood cells proved invaluable to scientists, including those at Pfizer, looking for new routes to preventing the spread of AIDS. Could they synthesize a molecule that would block the CCR-5 receptor on cells? And would that treatment mimic the state of those with natural HIV immunity, with a new medicine blocking the entry of the virus into the cell?

This hypothesis did not have universal acceptance. Some speculated that if the CCR-5 entry was blocked, HIV might find another entry into the cell. In fact, another such entry way has been uncovered called the CXCR-4 receptor, although this route appears to be rarely used by HIV. Would blockade of CCR-5 force the virus to use the second receptor? While the majority of strains of HIV bind through CCR-5, this question could not be answered until one tested a CCR-5 antagonist in patients. Once again, scientists had to invent a new molecule to be able to answer these questions.

THE IMPORTANCE OF HIGH-THROUGHPUT SCREENING

Pfizer scientists began a program to find a blocker of the CCR-5 receptor in 1996. They set up an assay that would measure a compound's ability to bind to the CCR-5 receptor and then proceeded to test over *one million* compounds for this activity over the next year. Such massive screening of compounds was unheard of in the 1980s. In those days, scientists could only manage to screen roughly 50 compounds per week in a given test. But that was before the invention of high throughput screening (HTS).

HTS was developed by two Pfizer scientists: Drs. John A. Williams and Dennis A. Pereira.[6] As part of the Molecular Genetics groups in 1984, they used molecular biology techniques to devise a method for screening fermentation broths as part of the hunt for novel antibiotics. Working with colleagues in Japan, they were able to automate their screening process such that 10,000 fermentation broths were screened weekly. Williams and Pereira recognized that this process could be adapted to the screening of small molecules as well and, by the mid-1980s, they had HTSs running for a number of Pfizer programs. These HTSs found a number of uniquely active molecules that propelled the advancement of a number of programs, thereby establishing HTS as a key tool in drug discovery. One of the many programs that used HTS was the CCR-5 program.

The discovery of HTS is another example of real innovation that pharmaceutical R&D brings in advancing medical science. In fact, HTS spawned a number of other innovations not just in screening compounds but also in the synthesis of compounds. By having HTS available, the bottleneck in the discovery of new medicines shifted to the availability of more compounds to screen. This led to automating chemical syntheses in such a way that huge libraries of compounds were able to be created. The principles of HTS were also applied to screening diverse biological assays such as P450 enzymes, protein binding, and general cytotoxicity. One could argue that contributions made by scientists like Williams and Pereira are greater than many other better recognized academic successes.

THE DISCOVERY OF SELZENTRY

Through HTS a key compound, UK-107,543, was found in 1997 that had activity of interest. This molecule was refined and modified, making changes to its structure, learning the impact of these changes on biological activity, and then making further refinements. At the end of 2000, a compound was singled out for further development: UK-427,857, generically known as maraviroc[7] (Figure 6.3). Early Phase 1 studies with maraviroc looked promising because it was a well-tolerated drug that had rapid and sustained blood levels to treat HIV.

A rapid reading on the efficacy of an anti-infectious agent in clinical trials can be relatively easily obtained in that the drug can be administered and blood samples can be taken to determine if the infectious agent is being killed. In the case of treating HIV, a patient's viral load can be measured. If the novel medicine is active, the patient's level of virus should drop. The first Phase 2 study with maraviroc generated a truly rewarding result. As shown in Figure 6.4, patients dosed with maraviroc at 100 mg twice a day for 14 days had roughly a 20-fold drop in their viral load. Placebo had no effect. As expected, once drug treatment stopped, the viral load returned to the original levels. This confirmed the original hypothesis: By blocking the CCR-5 receptor with a novel drug, one could mimic the situation resulting from the CCR5-Δ32 genetic mutation.

One cannot stress enough how exciting such a result was for the hundreds of scientists who had been involved up to this point. Over a period of more than seven years, these dedicated individuals set out to develop a totally new approach to treating AIDS. And now, they had the first evidence to show that it could work in people

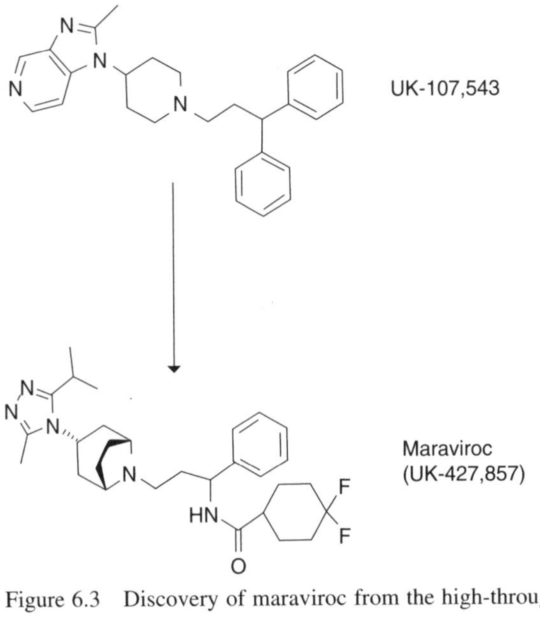

Figure 6.3   Discovery of maraviroc from the high-throughput screening hit, UK-107,453.

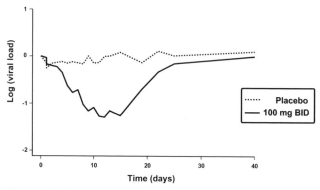

Figure 6.4   Reduction in viral load with Selzentry in HIV-positive patients.

with this dreaded disease. Dr. Patrick Dorr was a biologist on this program, and his memories from this time are quite telling.

> I vividly remember going to the 10th Conference on Retroviruses and Opportunistic Infections (CROI) in 2003 at Boston with the CCR-5 team to disclose our first data on maraviroc—then simply known as UK-427,857—a milestone. The disclosure followed favorable pharmacokinetics from first in human studies, and a great preclinical profile. At the time, I was swamped with writing study reports for Pfizer's CCR-5 candidate. I worked in the airport, on the plane, and in the hotel room upon arrival to try to meet the deadlines. I came close to ducking out of the introductory speeches at the conference to keep up the writing as I was not on schedule for completing the reports. However, I came to my senses and went along to the opening speeches. I think it was one of the best decisions of my career. The conference was opened by the Sinikithemba gospel choir from South Africa, all members of which were HIV positive. Their performance was beautiful. The choir leader was planning to give a speech to open the conference, but she was not well, and one of the choir members stood in for her. Her speech was the most moving I have ever heard. She described how becoming HIV positive resulted in her health declining until she was bed-ridden and was turning into a piece of meat. She had seen what AIDS had done to many of her friends, and was witnessing her family fall into deep poverty and suffering as she was the breadwinner, but did not have the health to move out of bed. She despaired. She explained that she counted herself as extremely lucky to get recruited into a clinical trial, and received anti-retroviral drugs. This reversed her fortunes. Her immune function and health returned, her working life returned, and her family moved out of poverty and began to thrive. She sincerely thanked the audience for their contribution in helping the fight against AIDS. She said she had never missed a dose of her antiretroviral drugs, did not care about the number of tablets, and that we should never lose sight of this. HIV resistance was scaring her, and she hoped we continued to look for additional new therapies to help her and the HIV positive world. She was one person amongst the millions infected and dying a horrible death. She kept thanking the audience—I was very humbled. She got a resounding standing ovation. Bill Clinton, who I have read is widely considered to be the finest speaker the world has seen, followed the gospel singer. If I was him I would have asked to have spoken first. I always counted myself very lucky to be part of the CCR-5 team. This made me feel proud to be working

against HIV, and to be associated with a promising program like maraviroc. I cannot put myself in the shoes of an HIV positive individual, but speeches like that help you better understand patient needs, and get you out of bed in the morning to go to work. Deadlines for study reports are no bad thing.

While promising, the Selzentry program was still a long way from the goal line.

The initial Phase 3 studies with maraviroc focused on AIDS patients whose treatments were beginning to become less efficacious due to viral resistance. These patients were running out of options. In this study, maraviroc, in combination with a patient's existing optimized treatment, was compared with patients on placebo and optimized therapy. The results proved very gratifying. In half of the patients that had maraviroc as part of their drug regimen, blood levels of HIV were undetectable. They once again were able to receive treatment to keep their disease in check. With these results in hand, the regulatory dossiers were filed in both Europe and the United States. Maraviroc was granted priority review by regulators on both sides of the Atlantic. On April 23, 2007, eleven years after beginning this program, an FDA Advisory Committee unanimously recommended accelerated approval for treatment-experienced patients. Maraviroc is now commercially available to these patients in the United States under the trade name Selzentry®. Selzentry[8] was the first new class of oral HIV therapy approved in a decade.

Scientific studies with Selzentry are continuing. Of great interest is the efficacy of this drug in newly diagnosed AIDS patients. Will a CCR-5 antagonist be equally effective as a first line of therapy? Clinical trials are underway to test this. But for now, a major medical advance has been made. For patients who have been living with AIDS for more than a decade and for whom the current benefits of their therapy are eroding, Selzentry offers hope for a continued high quality of life for years to come.

As was stated earlier, the uninformed would have associated a program like the CCR-5 project with the biotech industry. Obviously that is not the case. In fact the imaginary line between biotech and Big Pharma is blurring considerably. Companies like Amgen and Genentech are now larger than many pharmaceutical companies and are complementing their efforts in biologicals by building up expertise in small molecule drug discovery. Pfizer itself has publicly announced that it is ramping up efforts in the discovery and development of biologicals. The rational for this blurring is really quite simple. These companies are trying to bring medicines to patients. To treat diseases like cancer, Alzheimer's disease, or diabetes, a patient may need a medicine that could be a biologic or a pill. Patients want their disease to be controlled, if not cured. And these companies are in search of medical breakthroughs regardless of how they are packaged.

Here is one final bit of information that blurs this divide. At least one biotech company is vigorously pursing a next-generation small-molecule CCR-5 antagonist.[9] This shouldn't be a surprise. Both the biotech industry and Big Pharma have the same mission. Be it a first-in-class or a best-in-class medicine, each sector uses its resources to do this. There are no shortcuts: both face the same challenges and hurdles in discovering and developing new drugs. And, thankfully, innovation thrives in both worlds.

PART *III*

THE PROFIT MOTIVE

THE FIRST two parts of this book focused on how the pharmaceutical industry adds value in a number of ways, specifically how outstanding science is carried out to understand how best to treat diseases. This work involves tremendous innovation that produces new medicines that can save money for health care systems around the globe. Sadly, most industry critics don't recognize these contributions.

Some also assail the industry for all sorts of alleged sins. It is claimed that the industry invents diseases to foist unnecessary medications on the public. The industry is uncaring about the safety of its medicines. The industry tries to coerce patients and their physicians into utilizing these unsafe and unnecessary medications with misleading drug advertisements. The industry has no interest in people who cannot pay for these worthless medicines.

This section is meant to address an underlying concern that never quite emerges but is always in the background. Namely, that the profit motive in the pharmaceutical industry taints their work, the implication being that research results are manipulated or shaded to hide negative findings or to highlight only positive results. It is not unusual to hear a news report about a major new important drug study that concludes with: "But this study was funded by a pharmaceutical company." In other words, such results should not be trusted.

These accusations are ludicrous. No business could possibly survive if it behaved in such a manner. The next chapters will address each point to show what the facts truly are.

CHAPTER 7

THE INDUSTRY INVENTS DISEASES

T**HE HUNDREDS** of thousands of people in pharmaceutical R&D arrive at work each day with the hope and drive to discover and develop new medicines. They deeply believe in their work and their industry's mission. They recognize the difficult challenges they face, but also recognize that things that are truly worthwhile require hard work, diligence, and a bit of luck. While they do not expect to be treated like heroes, they certainly hope they deserve the support of the general public— or at least the support of people involved in health care. Unfortunately, this is not always the case as evidenced by the following excerpt from an article in the *British Medical Journal* entitled "Selling sickness: The pharmaceutical industry and disease mongering."[1]

> There's a lot of money to be made from telling healthy people they're sick. Some form of medicalising ordinary life may now be better described as disease mongering: widening the boundaries of treatable illness in order to expand markets for those who sell and deliver treatments. Pharmaceutical companies are actively involved in sponsoring the definition of diseases and promoting them to both prescribers and consumers. The social construction of illness is being replaced by the corporate construction of disease.

A cottage industry has been built upon the notion that the drug industry spends the bulk of its time working on unnecessary medicines. Here are just a few titles of books related to this topic[2a–c]:

> *Our Daily Meds: How the Pharmaceutical Companies Transformed Themselves into Slick Marketing Machines and Hooked the Nation on Prescription Drugs* by Melody Petersen
>
> *Overdosed America: The Broken Promise of American Medicine* by John Abramson
>
> *Over Dose: The Case Against the Drug Companies* by Jay Cohen

Judging from these sensationalized headlines, it appears that the pharmaceutical industry is the root of all evil.

Drug Truths: Dispelling the Myths About Pharma R&D, by John L. LaMattina
Copyright © 2009 John Wiley & Sons, Inc.

The view that the pharmaceutical industry sits around dreaming up new diseases and then convinces people that their minor ailment urgently needs drug treatment is absurd. First of all, a company cannot simply declare a new disease and market a drug to treat it. A disease must be recognized by global regulatory agencies who set up criteria that a drug must meet in order to have even the most remote chance to be approved. Second, payers must believe that the condition is serious enough to warrant reimbursement of the cost of the drug to treat it. Third, physicians must believe the disease is serious enough to be willing to prescribe a drug to their patient to treat it. And finally, patients must be concerned enough about their pain or discomfort to be willing to seek treatment in the first place. Thus, in order for the "world disease mongering conspiracy" to be successful, patients, physicians, payers, and regulators must act in concert with the exploitative drug companies. Doesn't this seem the least bit far-fetched?

Critics attack the pharmaceutical industry for turning conditions like "bone-thinning" and "hypercholesterolemia" into diseases. Is "bone-thinning" a disease? No. However, if you are a petite woman of Asian or Northern European descent, bone-thinning is the first sign of osteoporosis. Should you wait until your bones are brittle or even breaking before starting drug treatment? No, because by then it will be too late. Similarly, if you are an overweight male with high LDL cholesterol and have a family history of heart disease and if diet and exercise have not been enough to control your cholesterol levels, should you take a statin? Given that statin use lowers your risk of a heart attack by as much as 35%, the answer should be a resounding "yes"! This type of treatment is not disease mongering—it is preventative medicine.

A frequent target of the "disease mongering" attackers is a condition known as irritable bowel syndrome (IBS). On the surface this sounds like an innocuous problem. However, a person with IBS has the following symptoms: abdominal pain, a feeling of bloating, and alteration of bowel habits that can be either diarrhea predominant (IBS-D) or constipation predominant (IBS-C). This is not a life-threatening condition. However, IBS symptoms impact a person's quality of life, because it affects sleep, diet, ability to travel, and sexual function. Patients are concerned enough about it that the largest percentage of referrals to gastroenterologists is due to IBS.[3] The cost of IBS treatment in the United States is estimated to be between $1.7 billion and $10 billion in direct medical costs, *excluding* prescription and over-the-counter drug costs. This is clearly not a disease invented by a pharmaceutical sales executive.

It is easy for critics to accuse companies of inventing fictitious diseases to increase sales. In a world plagued with AIDS, Alzheimer's disease, and cancer, something like IBS can seem unimportant—unless you suffer from it. For adolescents with severe acne, their own condition can leave both physical and emotional scars. They too don't consider their own condition too trivial for medical research. People suffering from a specific ailment, be it called a syndrome, a condition, or a disease, will seek out treatment if their quality of life is restricted by their ailment.

As was stated above, a pharmaceutical company cannot simply declare that a new disease exists and begin marketing a product to treat it. A company must get approval from regulatory agencies to market a drug for a new indication, and this process is as vigorous as that for a new drug to treat an established disease such as diabetes. To understand how this process works, two examples will be discussed: Zoloft to treat post-traumatic stress syndrome (PTSD) and Lyrica to treat fibromyalgia.

ZOLOFT® AND PTSD

PTSD is an anxiety disorder that is characterized by fear, helplessness, or horror in a person who has been exposed to a major traumatic event. This event can range from experiencing violence on a personal level, such as witnessing a violent injury or unnatural death, to being exposed to a major event such as the terrorist attack on the World Trade Center on September 11, 2001. Such events precipitate a variety of responses in PTSD patients, which include: (a) re-experiencing the event through nightmares and flashbacks; (b) avoidance of people and places associated with the incident as well as amnesia; and (c) hyper-arousal resulting in insomnia, exaggerated startle reactions and impaired concentrations.[4] A complete list of the diagnostic criteria for PTSD appears in Figure 7.1. As can be seen, this is a very serious disorder.

The harmful effects of traumatic events on individuals have been known for years. Horowitz[5] helped to conceptualize the idea of this being a general syndrome in 1976, and in 1980 the American Psychiatric Association codified this as PTSD. PTSD is commonly associated with combat veterans, having been popularized as "battle fatigue" or "shell shock." However, women are twice as likely to suffer PTSD as men. This is because interpersonal violence is a major driver for PTSD. PTSD develops in 55% of rape victims compared to 2% of those involved in a major disaster. It is not clear whether the higher prevalence rates in women are the results of women being more susceptible to PTSD or whether the rates of sexual and physical assaults on women are much higher than for men.[4]

In the late 1990s, PTSD was treated largely by psychotherapy. There were no drugs approved for PTSD. However, there was reason to believe that the selective serotonin reuptake inhibitor (SSRI) antidepressants might be of value for treating PTSD because clinical pharmacology studies suggested that the central serotonergic neuronal systems play a role in PTSD. Furthermore, there were anecdotal examples reported in the literature showing that SSRIs were efficacious in alleviating the avoidance and numbing symptoms of PTSD. Unfortunately, there were no validated animal models of PTSD to test this hypothesis. To prove or disprove the theory that an SSRI would be of value to treat PTSD, clinical trials needed to be carried out. So Pfizer scientists consulted the FDA about using Zoloft (generic name, sertraline) in treating PTSD patients. This meeting was a critical step in this process. Because no drug had been approved for PTSD, having the FDA's views on what type of studies were needed, what criteria should be measured, how long the studies should be conducted, and so on, were crucial in order to perform a valid test of this concept that would be acceptable to regulatory agencies and to payers as proof of Zoloft's efficacy. The FDA predetermines what parameters should be measured in patients and what outcomes will be needed for approval. These guidelines are set before a

A person must have been exposed to a traumatic event.
 The event involved a perceived or actual threat to the person's own life or physical integrity or that of another, such as a physical or sexual assault, rape, a serious accident, a natural disaster, combat, being taken hostage, torture, displacement as a refugee, sudden unexpected death of a loved one, and witnessing a traumatic event.
 The person's response to the event involved fear, helplessness, or horror.
The person persistently experiences the event in at least one of several ways:
 The person has intrusive recollections of the event.
 The person has nightmares.
 The person has flashbacks, which are particularly vivid memories that occur while he or she is awake and make him or her act or feel as though the event was recurring.
 The person has intense psychological distress in response to reminders of the traumatic event.
 The person has intense physiological reactions in response to reminders of the event (including palpitations, sweating, difficulty breathing, and other panic responses).
The person avoids reminders of the event and has generalized numbness of feeling, as indicated by the presence of at least three of the following:
 The person actively avoids pursuits, people, and places that remind him or her of the event.
 The person avoids thinking of or talking about the event.
 The person is unable to recall aspects of the event.
 The person has lost interest in or participates less in activities.
 The person has felt detached or estranged from other people since the event.
 The person has a restricted range of emotions or a feeling of numbness.
 The person feels as though his or her life has been foreshortened or as though there is no need to plan for the future, with respect to his or her career, getting married, or having children.
The person has symptoms of increased arousal, as evidenced by the presence of at least two of the following:
 The person has difficulty falling or staying asleep (sometimes related to fear of having nightmares).
 The person is irritable and has feelings or outbursts of anger.
 The person has difficulty concentrating.
 The person has become more vigilant and concerned about safety.
 The person has exaggerated startle reactions in response to sounds or movements.
The three types of symptoms must be present together for at least one month.
The disorder must cause clinically significant distress or impairment in social, occupations, or other areas of functioning.

Figure 7.1 Diagnostic criteria for PTSD. There are three subtypes of PTSD. Acute PTSD refers to symptoms that last less than 3 months. Chronic PTSD refers to symptoms that last 3 months or longer. Delayed-onset PTSD refers to symptoms that begin at least 6 months after a traumatic event. Adapted from the *Diagnostic and Statistical Manual of Mental Disorders*, 4th edition. Copyright © 2002 Massachusetts Medical Society. All rights reserved.

single patient is studied and, if these guidelines are not met, the FDA will reject the clinical trials and the drug will not be approved.

An advantage of using Zoloft to validate the SSRI-PTSD hypothesis was that it was already a well-established, widely prescribed antidepressant. Millions of patients had already benefited from this medicine. Its safety was understood, it would be given once a day, and it did not interact badly with alcohol. Thus, it was an ideal compound to use to test the hypothesis that an SSRI would benefit people suffering with PTSD.

Studies began in 1996. Patients who had a minimum duration of 6 months of PTSD were dosed with either Zoloft or placebo over 12 weeks. Both patients and doctors were unaware of which treatment the patients were getting (a "double blind study"). Because of the marked impairment in occupational, health and psychosocial functioning associated with PTSD, the trial was designed to assess not only symptomatic outcomes but also psychosocial and quality of life outcomes as well. PTSD has been characterized as one of the most functionally debilitating disorders known. Even small symptom improvements that lead to resumed daily activities as simple as driving or taking elevators can have a meaningful impact on family and work life. At the start of the study patients were assessed using standardized questionnaires that had been previously developed by experts in the field.[6]

For regulatory approval, positive, statistically significant results from two well-controlled clinical trials were required. This is to ensure that the benefits seen are indeed real and will translate to the general population. Gratifyingly, two such studies were achieved with Zoloft in PTSD patients. In the first, patients had a 60% responder rate on Zoloft compared to 38% on placebo[7]; the second showed a 53% responder rate on Zoloft compared to 32% on placebo.[8] These studies showed that after 12 weeks, patients on Zoloft improved on measures of social relationships, leisure activities, ability to function daily, living situation, ability to get around physically, and ability to work. In short, it restored a more normal life.

While both of these studies were carried out in a general population of PTSD patients, in fact 80% of the patients were female. As stated earlier, this predominance of females in this study is not surprising given that women make up the bulk of the population for this syndrome. Another study was also run with the Veterans Administration looking at those who had served in a war zone with PTSD resulting from exposure to combat related trauma.[9] The same design was used for this study as compared to the ones described earlier. In this patient population, which was almost 80% male, it was disappointing to find that Zoloft offered no benefit over placebo. It was unclear as to why combat veterans did not benefit from SSRI treatment. Male patients in VA settings have an especially long duration of illness and so perhaps PTSD is more established and more difficult to treat in this patient population. Nevertheless, Zoloft is not effective in treating PTSD in a VA setting despite its proven efficacy in the civilian population.

Armed with the results of these studies, the Pfizer team filed a New Drug Application (NDA) with the FDA for a new use for Zoloft in the treatment of PTSD. Because no drug had been approved for PTSD, the FDA's Division of Neuropharmacological Drug Products (the division is responsible for approving Central Nervous System drugs) convened an Advisory Committee (AC) meeting to judge the merits of the NDA. The Committee is made up of leading physicians and scientists in a particular field, and each division of the FDA has such standing committees. The FDA will often solicit their advice on a variety of topics, especially when a drug of a new mechanistic class or a drug for a new disease indication is being considered. While the FDA is not required to accept the recommendation of an advisory committee, it frequently does.

In October 1999, the Psychopharmacologic Drug Advisory Committee met to discuss the application for the use of Zoloft to treat PTSD. They were asked by the FDA to answer the following questions:

1. Has the sponsor (Pfizer) provided evidence from more than one adequate and well-controlled clinical investigation that supports the conclusion that Zoloft is effective for the treatment of PTSD?

2. Has the sponsor provided evidence that Zoloft is safe when used in the treatment of PTSD?

At the end of the day-long series of presentations, discussions, and debate, the Advisory Committee voted 6–1 in favor of question one and 7–0 in favor of question two. In December 1999, the FDA formally approved the first drug to treat PTSD, Zoloft. Of course, no one at that time had ever envisioned the events of 9/11. Thankfully, however, in 2001 there was a treatment available to help patients with the ensuing trauma caused on that horrible day.

LYRICA® AND FIBROMYALGIA

Imagine waking up from surgery and finding that, while the operation took care of your immediate problem, you now had something new and insidious—a syndrome called fibromyalgia. This is exactly what happened to Ms. Lynne Matallana.[10] In 1993 after uterine surgery, she had pain throughout her body. She couldn't wear jewelry because it hurt her skin. Even bed sheets were painful to her feet. She saw 37 doctors, but the pain never went away. She was eventually diagnosed with fibromyalgia and she became a crusader against this condition, becoming the co-founder and president of the National Fibromyalgia Association.

Fibromyalgia is not a new disease. Clinical descriptions of it have appeared for over 150 years.[10] Characterized by widespread pain that can be relentless, fibromyalgia is usually accompanied by poor sleep, stiffness, and fatigue. Sufferers also experience deep soreness/tenderness and flu-like aching. The pain of fibromyalgia can hamper a patient's ability to work and often results in increased medical costs and disability.

The cause of fibromyalgia is unknown, but its onset is often attributed to a stressful event such as major surgery, infection, or trauma. In addition, genetic factors may predispose people to fibromyalgia. This is a very common condition that is estimated to affect approximately 2% of the adult population in the United States and is far more prevalent in women (3.4%) than in men (0.5%).[11] Before 2007, there was no treatment for fibromyalgia approved by the FDA or the European Regulatory Agency. Because of the multiple symptoms present in fibromyalgia, pharmaceutical companies struggled to devise a single effective treatment for this condition.

Fibromyalgia was thought to result from neurological changes in how patients perceive pain, specifically a heightened sensitivity to stimuli that are not normally painful. Interestingly, Pfizer had an agent already on the market, Lyrica (generic name: pregabalin), that was known to bind to a specific protein within overexcited nerve cells. As a result, it helped to calm damaged nerves. Lyrica had already been approved to treat such painful conditions as neuropathy resulting from diabetes and also post-herpetic neuralgia. Pfizer scientists believed that Lyrica could also be effective in treating the neural pain associated with fibromyalgia.

As was the case with Zoloft and PTSD, meetings were held with the FDA in 2004 to design clinical studies that would be acceptable in demonstrating the effectiveness of Lyrica in treating fibromyalgia. The clinical studies were carried out in 2005 and 2006, with the results filed with the FDA in December 2006. As with Zoloft, Lyrica was already on the market for other indications, millions of patients had been exposed to it around the world, and the safety of this medicine was understood. The key question that had to be answered in the fibromyalgia clinical program was pretty basic: did Lyrica relieve the pain and symptoms of fibromyalgia?

The answer proved to a resounding "yes." In one study depicted in Figure 7.2, Lyrica provided rapid relief of chronic widespread pain in fibromyalgia patients with significant effects being seen in the very first week of dosing. These results are from a 14-week randomized, double-blind, placebo-controlled study of 745 patients that evaluated the safety and efficacy of Lyrica. The primary efficacy measure was symptomatic relief of pain associated with fibromyalgia.

Not only was the pain relief rapid, it also proved to be durable as well. The FREEDOM (Fibromyalgia Relapse Evaluation and Efficacy for Durability of Meaningful Relief) trial demonstrated significant long-term pain improvement in patients with fibromyalgia for up to 6 months.[12] This double-blind, placebo-controlled study involved 1051 patients with fibromyalgia. During the first phase, all patients received Lyrica and were asked to evaluate their response to therapy. At the end of 6 weeks, more than 50% reported a reduction in pain and being "much" or "very much" improved. In the second phase, 556 patients who had responded to Lyrica were

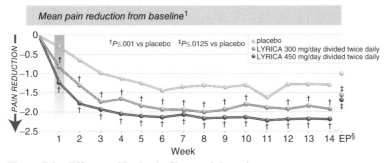

Figure 7.2   Efficacy of Lyrica in fibromyalgia patients.

randomly assigned to receive continued treatment or given placebo for 6 months. Pain relief was maintained in nearly twice as many patients treated with Lyrica (68%) compared to those who were switched to placebo (39%).

Because of the major medical need that existed for a treatment of fibromyalgia, the FDA gave the NDA for the Lyrica fibromyalgia indication "Priority Review" status. The FDA gave its approval on June 22, 2007. For the first time, fibromyalgia patients had an approved drug for this debilitating condition. One such fibromyalgia patient, Carolyn Bishop, said the following about the success she had with Lyrica for her condition:

> I couldn't spend time with my kids and do the things that I wanted to do with them. You know, I went from being able to hike and bike and walk around and go shopping and go to the movies and hang out with my friends. I could not even get off of the sofa for three days at a time. Within two weeks after reaching my dosage level, I started having a life again. I got to go out with my family. I got to have lunch with friends. I went to a movie, which was something I had not been able to do because it hurt so bad to sit in a theater chair.

All those patients who had been told that their "disease was in their head" or that nothing could be done for their condition could now experience substantial relief.

There are obvious similarities between the two examples just discussed: Zoloft for PTSD and Lyrica for fibromyalgia. Both PTSD and fibromyalgia had been known for decades. Yet both were poorly defined, poorly understood, and poorly treated. Physicians were unable to treat these conditions easily; and patients were not only frustrated, but suffered at the lack of treatment options. In the worst-case situation, their conditions were ignored or even trivialized.

Pfizer had medicines already available and used by patients to treat other diseases. For both PTSD and fibromyalgia, there were scientific theories that Zoloft for the former and Lyrica for the latter would provide much needed relief for these conditions. The FDA determined what studies were required to demonstrate safety and efficacy. Is this "disease mongering"? Is this "medicalizing ordinary life"? Is this "corporate construction of disease"? Those patients whose lives have been changed by Zoloft and Lyrica dismiss such absurd accusations.

CHAPTER 8

NEW DRUGS ARE LESS SAFE
THAN TRADITIONAL MEDICINES

HOW DIFFICULT is it to discover and develop a medicine that would be universally safe and effective in millions and millions of patients around the world? Actually, it is more than difficult—it is virtually impossible. It is unreasonable to expect that one pill would have identical effects in the young or old, male or female, large or small, and all members of different racial and ethnic groups. Think about people with peanut allergies who can die by ingesting a single nut, or others who are lactose-intolerant. If basic foods aren't tolerated by all, how can it be expected that a medicine should behave identically in all who need it?

That doesn't mean, however, that the pharmaceutical industry has a cavalier attitude when it comes to the safety of new medicines and the patients who take them. Quite the opposite is true. And yet, this is questioned by many. In the article "List of Problem Prescription Drugs is Growing,"[1] Mr. Arthur Levin, Director of the Center for Medical Consumers states:

> In recent history there has been increasing pressure to get new drugs to market, and that comes from a lot of sectors: patients and their organizations, the drug companies and, of course, people in Congress who think the FDA gets in the way of drugs reaching the marketplace.

The implication in this statement is that the rapid approval of a new medicine results in a less than rigorous review of its credentials. This is not true. Yet, Levin's point provides food for thought. There is a desire on a lot of fronts to get important new medicines to patients. However, the hurdles to get a new drug approved by the FDA and other regulatory agencies around the world are higher than ever. So where is the disconnect?

As has been described in an earlier chapter, when a New Drug Application is submitted, in general 5000 to 20,000 patients will have been treated with the new medicine. Every patient who has been part of these studies has had their medical records thoroughly reviewed by the company filing the NDA, by the hospitals and clinics that have tested the experimental medicine and by the FDA. Assuming the data in the dossier demonstrate the safety and efficacy of the new medicine, it will be approved for general use. However, at this point it has been studied in just thousands of patients. One might ask whether the FDA should require that the

---

experimental agent be tested in perhaps as many as 100,000 patients before approval. Given the enormous costs and the lengthy time involved currently in bringing a new medicine to market, such a ramp up in clinical studies would prohibit all further drug development.

This does not mean, however, that a sponsor is done with patient safety monitoring once it receives an NDA approval. In fact, a company is responsible for identifying, analyzing, and reporting to regulatory agencies potential safety issues at every point in the life of a medicine for as long as it is prescribed by physicians. Many, many scientists are employed by each pharmaceutical company to monitor adverse events of marketed drugs. Using information reported by physicians, patients, and caregivers, they try to detect health risks and emerging safety signals as soon as possible, and they must report them to the FDA and other regulatory agencies around the world.

Once millions of patients have been exposed to a new medicine, it can be viewed differently. As was described in Chapter 5, it wasn't until Chantix had been prescribed to millions of smokers that suicidal ideation was noted in a very small percentage of users. Companies and regulators must constantly weigh emerging risks against the established benefits of the product and, in this instance, it was determined that the benefits of Chantix far outweighed the risks. Nevertheless, in consultation with the FDA, the label for Chantix was altered to reflect this concern and to make patients and physicians aware of this so that those on this drug can be monitored for behavior and mood changes.

There are times, however, when such broad utilization of a medication can identify unexpected risk that does, in fact, result in the medicine being pulled from the marketplace. An example of this will be presented later in this chapter. This type of discontinuation is certainly concerning, but it demonstrates that the system works. As stated at the outset, no medicine is without risk, nor are we likely to identify all possible risks in a database of several thousand patients.

It is important that, when safety signals are seen with new drugs, these get properly communicated broadly to patients and physicians. The resulting publicity unfortunately gives the impression that all new medicines are inherently risky and that older medicines are safer. There is also the perception that over-the-counter (OTC) medications are benign. This is not the case. One of the scarier examples of the dangers of misusing OTC drugs was reported recently in the *New England Journal of Medicine*.[2] This perspective addressed the use of cough and cold medications in children. The authors reported that six studies exploring the use of these remedies in children under 12 years of age found that these drugs had no more activity than placebo. More concerning, however, was not the lack of efficacy but rather the potential danger in the use of such so-called remedies. The authors cited a recent report from the Centers for Disease Control and Prevention that showed that 1500 emergency room visits were recorded in 2004 and 2005 for children less than 2 years of age who had been given cough and cold products. Basically, every 12 hours a baby is sent to an emergency room in the United States as a result of being given an ineffective cough or cold product. One can only imagine the headlines that such a finding would create if this was due to a new prescription medication!

The potential toxicity of commonly used OTC medications extends to adults as well. Again, there is a sense that if you buy something in your neighborhood supermarket it must be very safe. Yet, the number one cause of liver failure in the United States is available on these same shelves. Overdose of acetaminophen, the active ingredient of Tylenol, is the leading cause for calls to Poison Control Centers (>100,000 per year). This medicine accounts for more than 56,000 emergency room visits, 2600 hospitalizations, and an estimated 458 deaths annually as a result of acute liver failure.[3] Acetaminophen taken in recommended dosages is safe. It is metabolized in the liver, and no health issues arise as long as a patient's liver is healthy. However, if the liver is overwhelmed with a large amount of acetaminophen or if the liver is already damaged because of infection or alcohol abuse, abnormal metabolism of acetaminophen can occur, thereby producing lethal byproducts. The majority of acetaminophen overdoses occur as a result of suicide attempts.

Does this mean that this OTC pain medication should be removed from super-market shelves? Of course not. However, this is yet another example of the risk–benefit balance that exists for every drug that one takes. In the case of acetaminophen, the benefits certainly predominate, but a patient must heed any and all precautions. The same is obviously true for prescription medicines.

Acetaminophen is not the only OTC pain reliever that can cause toxic reactions. In an article entitled "Take Two Possibly Lethal Pills and Call Me in the Morning," David Stipp describes a medicine that is "… commonly given to patients for non-fatal conditions such as mild inflammation. Yet, studies suggest that it and several drugs like it are fatal to at least 10,000 Americans a year. The victims die grisly deaths, typically from internal bleeding."[4] This drug is acetylsalicylic acid, also known as aspirin. This drug has been available for over a century and has prob-ably been ingested by over a billion people. And yet if it was discovered in a phar-maceutical R&D laboratory today, it would never have been developed. The reason for this is simple. In the standard animal testing models such as rats and dogs, gastric lesions and bleeding are observed very quickly. Such toxicity would never be accept-able by companies nor regulators for a new medicine becuase it would lead to thousands of patients being hospitalized from gastrointestinal bleeding. Thus, the scientists would abandon aspirin and look for a safer compound that provided pain relief without this toxicity. In fact, this is the very rationale for COX-2 inhibitors.

THE DISCOVERY OF COX-2 INHIBITORS

Aspirin is a member of a broad class of drugs known as nonsteroidal anti-inflammatory agents (NSAIDs). The compounds are distinguished by their ability to reduce inflammation. Inflammation is a response by the immune system to a chal-lenge or insult such as nerve damage or infection. Inflammation is characterized by pain, redness, swelling, warmness, and, depending on the site, a loss of mobility. Over the past decades, a number of different types of traditional NSAIDs have been invented and marketed. These include such commonly used agents as ibuprofen and naproxen. The proliferation of traditional NSAIDs is due to a variety of reasons, but two stand out. First, scientists have always sought a "safer aspirin," one without the gastrointestinal effects and other liabilities that aspirin brings. The second reason is one that is fundamental to the management of pain. Pain is a very heterogeneous condition, one that is poorly understood. As a result, management of pain can be challenging for patients and physicians. Medicines that work wonders for some people with arthritis may do nothing for others. In fact, new pain medications sell rapidly soon after they are launched because people with poorly controlled pain, unrelieved with existing analgesics, are anxious to try something new. They hope that their overall quality of life will improve. Pain management is definitely an area where having multiple options greatly benefits the patient.

Traditional NSAIDs represent many different compounds from a molecular standpoint. However, all share a common characteristic: they inhibit the enzymes cyclooxygenase 1 and 2 (COX-1 and COX-2). These two enzymes are important in the body's production of a family of compounds known as prostaglandins, which are mediators that are ubiquitous in humans. (One aspect of prostaglandin activity has been previously discussed in Chapter 4.) Interestingly, it wasn't until the late 1980s that scientists recognized that there were at least two forms of cyclooxygenase.[5a,b] (In 2002, yet another form, COX-3, was identified!)[5c] More importantly, while they catalyze the same biochemical reaction, COX-1 and COX-2 proved to be quite different. COX-1, by nature of its broad presence in issue and organs, is largely responsible for the synthesis of certain prostaglandins that protect the stomach lining. Thus, when a traditional NSAID is used to treat pain and inflammation, it blocks the production of agents that maintain the integrity of the stomach lining, thereby facilitating gastrointestinal damage.

On the other hand, COX-2 levels are normally low. However, when tissue damage occurs, COX-2 is produced at the site of inflammation. COX-2 catalyzes the formation of proinflammatory prostaglandins and is considered to be an "inducible" enzyme—that is, one which is produced by various stimuli of inflammation. This information was an incredible revelation to scientists seeking novel anti-inflammatory agents. Understanding the role of COX-2 suggested a route to agents that could effectively mediate pain but do so without the side effects, particularly gastrointestinal ulceration. Many believed that a selective COX-2 inhibitor would provide excellent pain relief without the traditional NSAID side-effect baggage and thus provide a valuable new drug to treat arthritis and other painful conditions. The race was on.

One of the pioneers in the COX-2 field was Dr. Philip Needleman. Dr. Needleman spent 25 years at Washington University School of Medicine, where he rose to Professor and Chairman of the Department of Pharmacology. It was here that his work in COX-2 began. In fact, he coined the term "COX-2" because others had originally referred to this enzyme as a prostaglandin synthase. In 1989, he moved to industry, starting as a Senior Vice-President of Monsanto and then becoming the President of Searle R&D in 1993. With Searle's merger with Pharmacia, he assumed the role of Pharmacia's Chief Scientist in 2000, which he held until his departure in 2003.

Dr. Needleman continued to investigate COX-2 research at Searle, and this program was begun in earnest in 1991. Realizing the intense competition that was developing in this arena, he set a strategy to be "First to Market" and staffed this program aggressively. Early on, this program was staffed with 40 medicinal chemists, an enormous commitment especially considering the relative size of Searle's R&D group as compared to others. The key to success was getting a viable "lead"—a compound that demonstrated a degree of selectivity for COX-2 over COX-1. Searle scientists were drawn to a report by DuPont scientists that showed that an experimental compound, DuP-697, had good anti-inflammatory properties in rats but was devoid of the ulcergenic activity normally associated with indomethacin.[6] The Searle scientists tested DuP-697 and found it was in fact selective for COX-2 over COX-1. They then set out to improve upon this compound in order to identify a compound worthy enough to do clinical trials. Over the course of 1992 and 1993, Searle's medicinal chemists synthesized more than 2500 compounds, 280 of which met the necessary potency criteria. Eventually, seven were selected for full evaluation in animals which included toxicology studies, pharmacokinetic profiling, stability studies, and work on formulating these compounds into pills.

This was a very exciting time for these scientists. Dr. Karen Seibert was the head pharmacologist for this program. She had been a post-doctoral researcher in the Needleman laboratories at Washington University in 1988 and moved with him to Searle. Karen described the atmosphere at the time as follows.

> I remember sitting in a small think tank group every week, looking at early data form various leads, immersed in the excitement of the moment. Senior managers and scientists alike were there—but there was no "management" in that room, no hierarchy. The environment was seamless, authentic, committed. There was a level of "intimacy" among us. Everybody was rowing the boat together. The goal was set and NEVER changed. This would be our "man on the moon"—we would be FIRST with an important, hypothesis-driven new medicine in our field.

Interestingly, one of the seven compounds that was being advanced from the first cohort was indeed Celebrex® (generic name: celecoxib). However, Celebrex didn't stand out as a "eureka." Rather it wasn't until all of the advanced preclinical studies were done that it was selected for advancement into human studies and even then it was a close call with another compound. Searle began this program in August 1991, and in March 1995 the first volunteer was dosed with Celebrex in Phase 1.

The big moment came when the first pain data became available. Remember it was still only hypothetical that a COX-2 inhibitor would be as potent a pain reliever as a traditional NSAID; some even believed that both COX-1 and COX-2 inhibition was needed for pain relief. And it was also hypothetical that a selective COX-2 inhibitor would be better tolerated in the human GI tract. Celebrex showed significant pain relief from the very first study. The hope that pain alleviation would occur by blocking only COX-2 was realized. In addition, early gastrointestinal toleration data also supported the hypothesis that COX-2 inhibition would do little harm to the gastrointestinal tract.[7] Data from a study depicting both activities are shown in Figure 8.1. At this point the possibility that a COX-2 inhibitor could become a major new medicine became very real.

The extraordinary focus that Searle put into the discovery program carried into the development program as well. "At risk" investments of R&D funds were made early in the program even before the COX-2 hypothesis was validated with Celebrex.

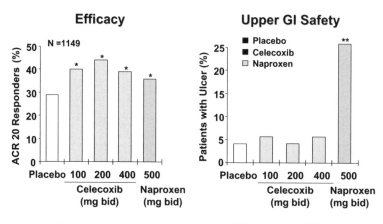

Figure 8.1   Celebrex efficacy and GI safety data.

For example, clinical supplies were prepared well in advance of the Phase 3 program. In addition, the Phase 2 program was streamlined and focused. The team had been very optimistic that the COX-2 hypothesis would pan out and wanted to move to Phase 3 rapidly. The execution of the clinical program was excellent: from the testing of Celebrex in volunteers to the filing of the NDA took 39 months. And the NDA, which included more than 50 studies and almost 15,000 patients on Celebrex, was the largest dossier filed for an agent of this type. Figures 8.2a and 8.2b put these data into perspective. The former shows the vast difference in the data contained in the Celebrex NDA as compared to that of a traditional NSAID, Etodolac. Not only were there more clinical trials in the Celebrex NDA, there were six times more patients on Celebrex than on Etodolac and the total exposure in patient-years was larger by 20-fold. In fact, the NDA for Celebrex had as many patients treated with this investigational drug as the NDAs for *six* previous traditional NSAIDs combined (Figure 8.2b).

The FDA had given Celebrex "Priority Review" status in recognition of the potential for this agent to be a significant improvement over traditional NSAIDs. It therefore received a 6-month accelerated review and was approved for marketing in December 1998. Searle had indeed landed their equivalent of a "man on the moon." While they were out in front, Searle was not alone. A month later, Merck received an approval for their COX-2 inhibitor, Vioxx® (generic name: rofecoxib). There were suddenly two alternatives to traditional NSAIDs for patients with arthritis.

THE POTENTIAL FOR COX-2 INHIBITORS IN TREATING COLON CANCER

In one of the very first conversations I had with Dr. Needleman, he expressed his vision for the COX-2 inhibitor field. He viewed this mechanistic class of agents as a technology platform and hoped that COX-2 inhibitors would be used for more

	Etodolac (1983)	Celecoxib (1998)
No. of Clinical Trials	40	51
No. of Patients	4,179	18,437
Placebo	1,036	2,450
Active Control	958	3,343
Study Drug	2,185	12,644
Single Dose	1,887	825
Multiple Doses	298	11,821
6 Month Treatment	158	2,429
1 Year Treatment	111	981
Total Exposure, Pt-Yrs	162	3,693

(a)

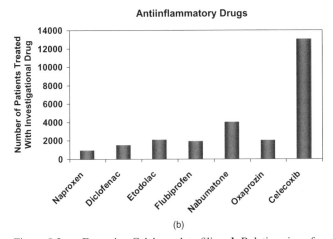

(b)

Figure 8.2   **a** Extensive Celebrex data filing. **b** Relative size of registration databases.

than pain, osteoarthritis, and rheumatoid arthritis. He had hopes that Celebrex might prove useful in other diseases such as cancer and that Celebrex might someday be more valued as an anticancer agent than as a "super aspirin." This vision was based on the fact that elevated levels of COX-2 are found in human tumor tissue samples, suggesting that COX-2 plays a role in tumor pathogenesis.

Even before the Celebrex clinical trials for arthritis had been completed, Searle had begun clinical studies with Celebrex in a condition known as Familial Adenomatous Polyposis (FAP). FAP is a rare genetic disease and progresses to colorectal cancer. People with FAP develop hundreds of polyps inside their large intestine. These polyps usually begin forming during puberty, and initial symptoms include diarrhea, stomach cramping, and bloody stools. If left untreated, these polyps will progress to colon cancer by the patient's third or fourth decade. FAP is treated with surgery but, since individual removal of each polyp is precluded, due to the very large number of polyps, surgeons remove the entire colon often with the rectum as well—a procedure that is both disfiguring and very debilitating. Patients with FAP have the choice of doing this in their early twenties or almost certainly getting colon cancer.

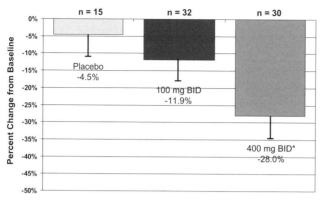

*p = 0.003 versus placebo

Figure 8.3   Percentage change from baseline in number of colorectal polyps (FAP patients).

These adenomatous colorectal polyps overexpress COX-2, and so it was hypothesized that inhibiting COX-2 production would result in regression of these polyps and reduce their progression to cancer. Therefore, a randomized, double-blind placebo-controlled trial was conducted to evaluate Celebrex in reducing the number and size of colorectal polyps in patients with FAP. The results are shown in Figure 8.3. This study demonstrated that Celebrex given at 400 mg twice a day was effective not only in significantly reducing the number of polyps but also in reducing polyp size and the percentage of patients whose disease progressed. Based on these results, in December 1999 the FDA approved a supplemental NDA for the use of Celebrex by FAP patients as an adjunct to the usual administered care.

The FAP results provided encouragement that COX-2 inhibitors could in fact be useful not just in this narrow patient population but perhaps also in broader groups as well. Thus, both Pfizer and Merck started long-term studies with their respective COX-2 inhibitors against colon cancer. Merck launched the "Adenomatous Polyp Prevention on Vioxx" (APPROVe) study, Pfizer began the "Prevention of Spontaneous Adenomatous Polyps" (Pre-SAP) trial, and the NIH started the "Adenoma Prevention with Celecoxib" (APC) trial. The fact that these studies were able to be done was a testament to the gastrointestinal safety that these COX-2 inhibitors demonstrated. Long-term studies of this ilk would have been difficult with traditional NSAIDs, given their gastrointestinal effects. Ironically, it was these studies that led to questions about the viability of the COX-2 inhibitor class.

CARDIOVASCULAR EFFECTS

On September 27, 2004, the Data Safety Monitoring Board for the APPROVe trial recommended that the study be stopped for safety reasons. The study showed an increased risk of cardiovascular events (including heart attack and stroke) in patients on Vioxx compared to placebo, particularly those who had been taking the drug for longer than 18 months.[8] The published data showed a dramatic inflection point in confirmed thrombotic events after this time versus placebo. Merck met with FDA officials on September 28 and informed the agency that they were voluntarily withdrawing Vioxx from the market. Merck had been concerned about the cardiovascular profile of Vioxx based on a previous study, the "Vioxx Gastrointestinal Outcomes Research" (VIGOR) program. While VIGOR demonstrated the gastrointestinal sparing effects of this COX-2 inhibitor, over the 1-year period of this study there were more cardiovascular events in the Vioxx arm than in the naproxen arm (there was no placebo arm in this study). The FDA was made aware of this result, and all subsequent Vioxx studies rigorously measured cardiovascular events.

The withdrawal of Vioxx from the market prompted people to question whether this toxicity was shared by other COX-2 inhibitors. Did this result apply to all members of this class of mechanism? At this time there were three long-term studies being conducted with the NIH that were ongoing for Celebrex: the two previously described, APC and Pre-SAP, along with a study looking at the potential use of Celebrex in treating Alzheimer's disease ("Alzheimer's Disease Anti-Inflammatory Prevention Trial," also known as ADAPT). The DSMB for the colon cancer studies had an independent cardiovascular subcommittee whose role was to monitor these trials for any signs of increased cardiac events. On December 16, 2004, the National Cancer Institute, which was sponsoring the APC trial, informed Pfizer that they were seeing an increased risk of fatal and nonfatal cardiovascular events in this trial. Analysis of the deaths due to heart attack, stroke, and heart failure after 3 years showed that there were 7 deaths out of 679 patients on placebo, 16 out of 685 patients on a daily dose of 400 mg of Celebrex, and 23 of 671 patients receiving a daily dose of 800 mg of Celebrex.[9] It should be noted that these doses were much higher than the usual dose to treat osteoarthritis, which is 200 mg or less per day.

Interestingly, the Pre-SAP trial that had been run for the same length of time and whose results were also monitored by the DSMB's cardiovascular subcommittee showed no evidence of cardiovascular risk. In Pre-SAP, there were cardiovascular-related deaths (1.8%) in 11 out of 628 patients on placebo as compared to 16 of 933 patients on 400 mg daily dose of Celebrex (1.7%). The safety monitoring group for the ADAPT trial also reviewed the cardiovascular event rate in this trial and found that in this patient population aged 70 and over with a family history of Alzheimer's disease, there were 28 deaths out of 717 patients on 400 mg daily of Celebrex (3.90%) as compared to 37 deaths of 1070 patients on placebo (3.46%)—essentially no difference. However, the traditional NSAID, naproxen, was also included in this trial and there were 40 cardiovascular related deaths of the 713 patients receiving 440 mg daily naproxen (5.61%).[10] In this study the COX-2 inhibitor proved benign, but the commonly used traditional NSAID demonstrated risk!

In light of all these confounding data, the investigators recommended the termination of all these studies, and this was done immediately. As a result, despite having invested over $100 million up to this point, the question as to whether Celebrex could indeed be of value in treating colon cancer or Alzheimer's disease was never answered.

FDA ADVISORY COMMITTEE MEETINGS

Suddenly, the FDA was confronted with a major dilemma. Given these results with both newer and older pain medications, how could they best advise the American populace on treating osteoarthritis, rheumatoid arthritis, and other painful conditions? The FDA convened a joint session of their Arthritis Advisory Committee and the Drug Safety and Risk Management Advisory Committee on February 16, 17, and 18, 2005. The FDA was seeking the advice of these experts as to whether these data supported a conclusion that increased cardiovascular risk is a class effect for all traditional NSAIDs, the COX-2 selective agents, or only certain agents within each class. The FDA also sought guidance on the risk–benefit balance for the COX-2 inhibitors.

This 3-day meeting had the elements of a courtroom drama. There was intense media interest from the major newspapers and television networks. About 300 people attended including those from drug companies, who were going to speak about their respective medicines, FDA experts to offer their views of these compounds, advocates both for and against the use of these drugs, and scientific experts in the field of arthritis, gastrointestinal disease, and cardiovascular disease. The audience even included investment analysts. The experts discussed their views of all the issues at hand: the relative safety of the COX-2 inhibitors in terms of gastrointestinal effects versus the older, traditional NSAIDs; the meaning of the data from the various colon cancer prevention studies; and the need for more studies to understand the cardiovascular effects of these drugs. One of the biggest surprises that emerged from these discussions was that there was indeed an increased risk of serious cardiovascular events with the traditional NSAIDs. This was found during a systematic review of observational studies from available databases and the scientific literature.[11a,b] Suddenly, all traditional NSAIDs at prescription doses were under scrutiny for adverse cardiovascular effects.

The Joint Advisory Committee digested and debated these data for 3 days, at the end of which they took a number of votes on questions provided by the FDA. Only a few are highlighted. The first two questions related to Celebrex. The FDA asked whether the available data supported the conclusion that Celebrex significantly increased the risk of cardiovascular events. The Joint Advisory Committee voted unanimously "yes" (32–0). However, on the question as to whether the risk versus benefit profile for Celebrex supported marketing in the United States, the Committee overwhelming voted "yes" by a 31–1 count, citing that they believed there was no risk at the 200-mg (arthritis) dose.

Despite the fact that Merck had already pulled Vioxx from the market, the FDA asked the Committee to vote as to whether Vioxx significantly increased the risk of cardiovascular events and then whether the risk–benefit profile supported its marketing in the United States. Again, the Committee voted unanimously on the first question but surprisingly voted 17–15 in favor of continued availability in the United States. It should be noted that many qualified their vote saying that only a low dose should be made available. Why did they vote this way? Perhaps they were moved by the testimony of a Vioxx patient. This woman had debilitating arthritis for years. None of the existing traditional NSAIDs, or even Celebrex, worked in controlling her pain. She described her life, largely confined to her home, unable to go out to visit friends or family due to her crippling condition. Then she tried Vioxx and her life changed. She started to remember what it felt to be "normal." She implored the Committee to allow Vioxx back on the market. She was unworried about any cardiovascular risk—she wanted to ease her pain. This story graphically illustrates how difficult it is to treat painful conditions and how drugs behave differently from one person to the next. Despite her plea and the Committee vote, Vioxx was never reintroduced to the market.

The Committee made a number of additional recommendations that related to Celebrex. They asked that a "black box" warning be added to the Celebrex label, as well as to the labels of all traditional NSAIDs. This was done, and for cardiovascular risk the black box warning read as follows:

> Celebrex may cause an increased risk of serious cardiovascular thrombotic events, myocardial infarction, and stroke, which can be fatal. All NSAIDs may have a similar risk. This risk may increase with duration of use. Patients with cardiovascular disease or risk factors for cardiovascular disease may be at greater risk.

The Committee, at the behest of the FDA, also made suggestions as to the design for a definitive study to compare the cardiovascular risk of COX-2 inhibitors, traditional NSAIDs, and placebo. There are more than 20 traditional NSAIDs approved for marketing in the United States and yet, unlike the situation for COX-2 inhibitors, no large long-term placebo-controlled trials had been conducted to evaluate long-term risks including cardiovascular risks. The reason for this was simple. Until the oncology studies were carried out with Vioxx and Celebrex, there was no reason to suspect such untoward effects of these older agents. It wasn't until the results of studies like APPROVe, APC, and ADAPT were available that there was a reason to go back through existing databases to see if there may be adverse cardiovascular signals with traditional NSAIDs. These observational studies are not conclusive, however. What is really needed is a long-term clinical trial to assess rigorously the potential cardiovascular effects of these drugs.

Based on the input of the Joint Advisory Committee, the FDA worked with Pfizer to design such a study. The result of this is PRECISION: "Prospective Randomized Evaluation of Celebrex Integrated Safety vs. Ibuprofen or Naproxen." This $300 million trial is being coordinated by the esteemed Cleveland Clinic, but it is sponsored by Pfizer. Clinical investigators will compare Celebrex (100–200 mg twice daily), ibuprofen (600–800 mg three times daily) and naproxen (375–500 mg twice daily) in patients with osteoarthritis or rheumatoid arthritis who are at risk of developing cardiovascular disease and who require one of these medications to control their arthritis symptoms. The primary endpoint for this study is the first occurrence of cardiovascular deaths, heart attack, and strokes, but other outcomes such as pain relief and the occurrence of significant gastrointestinal events will be measured as well. This study involves 20,000 patients and is scheduled for completion in December 2010.[12]

So how is a physician supposed to treat their patients in the wake of this pain medication crisis? An excellent perspective was provided in the *New England*

Journal of Medicine by Dr. Nancy J. Olsen, a professor of Arthritis at the University of Texas Southwestern Medical Center.[13] Dr. Olsen described some different patient situations and makes the following point:

> As these instances demonstrate, there are enough factors to be weighed in the choice of an arthritis medication that the risks and benefits ought to be considered on a case-by-case basis by a physician who knows the patient.

Until the results of PRECISION are available, this is clearly the most prudent approach in managing these patients.

THE SAFETY OF NEW DRUGS

It should be clear after reading this chapter that more is known about the drugs being developed today than at any time previously. There are good reasons for this. There is a great deal more understood about human physiology and the impact of new medicines on complex biological processes. In addition, more is understood about drug–drug interactions as well as about how the human body metabolizes new compounds. As a result, the FDA rightfully demands more studies of new drugs than ever before in order to understand the risk–benefit profile of these new potential medicines. The bar to regulatory approval is also higher than ever before. However, it must be noted that the bar was much lower when many commonly used medicines were first approved. This was not due to negligence—a lot less was understood about the long-term risk potential of drugs some years ago. Any medicine, be it aspirin, a cough medicine, or a newer medicine like Celebrex, needs to be used properly in order to avoid serious complications.

Karen Seibert has been with the Celebrex program from its earliest days. When asked about what were the most important moments for her in this program, she responded about the impact this drug had on those closest to herself and in doing so provided a wonderful perspective to close this story.

> One of my sisters has rheumatoid arthritis. She had suffered seriously with her disease—she had "walking on glass" symptoms that made it difficult to get to work, etc. Four days of naproxen always led to rectal bleeding. She entered the Celebrex Phase 3 trial and has been on it ever since and has had a life changing experience. Also, my husband has been able to manage completely his lower back pain with a combined Celebrex/Neurontin regimen. But I had another sister whose bed I stood next to for weeks as she was dying of cancer with poorly managed pain ... and I didn't have anything to offer her. This last memory humbles me and reminds me to this day that the work is not over; there are other needs of patients that we must satisfy.

CHAPTER 9

INDUSTRY SPENDS MORE
ON ADVERTISING THAN ON R&D

IN EARLY 2008, *USA Today* ran the following front page bold headlines:

As drug ads surge, more Rx's filled

This was the lead-in to a story reporting the results of a national survey of 1695 adults sponsored by *USA Today*, the Kaiser Family Foundation, and the Harvard School of Public Health.[1] The survey found that 32% of the respondents were prompted by prescription drug ads to ask their doctor about the medicine that was advertised, with 44% actually getting a prescription for the drug asked about. Interestingly, doctors recommended a different drug in 54% of the cases. The president of the Kaiser Foundation, Drew Altman, made the following observation:

> Our survey shows why the drug companies run all these ads: they work. Many people get drugs they otherwise wouldn't. While there is a debate about whether that's a good thing for patients, it does cost the country more.

This survey asked other questions including one on the amount of drug advertising that people are exposed to. In answer to the question "Do drug companies spend too much, too little, or about the right amount of money on advertising to patients?", 60% said "too much." An accompanying article alluded to advertising as a key factor in rising drug prices. There is a perception on the part of many that more is spent on advertising than on R&D and that, if pharmaceutical companies would spend less on commercials, drugs would be more plentiful and cheaper. What are the facts here?

Let's focus first on what the pharmaceutical industry actually spends on R&D. According to a report from the Congressional Budget Office,[2] "The pharmaceutical industry is one of the most research intensive industries in the United States." As shown in Figure 9.1, pharmaceutical companies invest five times more on R&D than the overall average for U.S. industries based on the percentage of annual sales in each sector.[3] Pharmaceutical companies invest significantly more in R&D than even research intensive enterprises such as software companies and aerospace/defense contractors. Furthermore, the pharmaceutical industry invests more than double what

Drug Truths: Dispelling the Myths About Pharma R&D, by John L. LaMattina
Copyright © 2009 John Wiley & Sons, Inc.

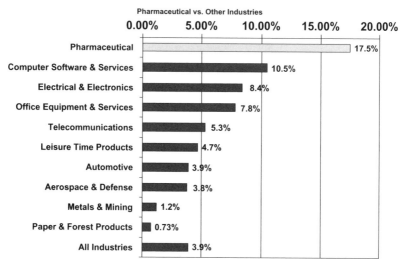

Figure 9.1   R&D expenditures as a percentage of annual revenues. (*Source*: PhRMA, 2006, based on data from PhRMA Annual Survey and Standard & Poor's Compustat, a division of McGraw-Hill.)

the National Institute of Health spends on R&D. In 2007, the NIH R&D budget was about $28 billion.[4] This compares to $58.8 billion of biopharmaceutical R&D expenditures.[5]

How does this investment in R&D compare to what industry spends on direct to consumer advertising (DTC)? First of all, DTC does not simply refer to television or radio advertisements. It also includes the promotion of prescription drugs through newspaper, magazine, and internet marketing as well. However, the whole topic of how drug companies not just advertise their products but also promote them is highly emotive. When discussing this, critics will state that all expenses incurred by the industry in the sale and marketing of their products include the costs for sales representatives, the value of drug samples given to physicians, and even the expenses for the corporate infrastructure of the marketing organization.[6a] Unfortunately, when the public hears "promotion of drugs," they often associate this directly with DTC expenditures. To confuse things further, estimates for these promotional costs fluctuate significantly. For this discussion, data will be used from an article in the *New England Journal of Medicine* that summarizes the DTC evolution of 1996–2005.[6b] In this paper, the authors provided information not just on DTC spending but also on overall promotional costs for prescription drugs. Figure 9.2 summarizes these costs for the 2001–2005 period. There is no doubt that DTC advertising has been going up from almost $3 billion in 2001 to $4.8 billion in 2006.[7] However, with worldwide prescription drug sales of approximately $600 billion, DTC advertising amounts to less than 1% of sales. Furthermore, the investment in R&D made by pharmaceutical companies is 10 times what is spent on DTC advertising.

What about the other promotional expenditures? What is noteworthy about the data reported in the *New England Journal of Medicine* (Figure 9.2) is that approxi-

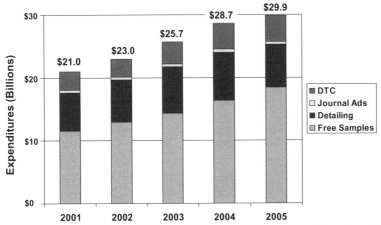

Figure 9.2   Breakdown on total promotional spending on prescription drugs 2001–2005.

mately 60% of the overall promotional spend by pharmaceutical companies is the value of free samples. These benefit both patients and physicians. For example, let's take a man who suffers from migraines and for whom older medications haven't worked well. Perhaps a sales representative has recently visited his physician to discuss a new migraine drug. The sales representative will usually leave the physician some free samples of the drug to try with her patients. On his next visit, the man's physician gives him some of these samples to see if it provides greater relief than his older medications. If the new drug works, the patient and the physician are both delighted and the man will get a prescription for the new drug. If the new drug is no better or perhaps even worse than his older treatment, he will naturally go back to his previous medicine. Does the pharmaceutical company hope that the patient will prefer its new medicine? Absolutely, and this is a proven way to generate interest in a new product. But the patient and physician both benefit as well since the patient tries a new drug for free and the physician gains first-hand experience with it.

If one were to include all promotional expenses in a given year, these costs are below the amount of money that pharmaceutical companies invest in R&D. These data are shown in Figure 9.3 for 2004 and 2005. As can be seen, even if the data in the *New England Journal of Medicine* article underestimated the promotional spending by $10 billion, the investment in R&D and promotional spending would be comparable. One can debate what the proper balance of the R&D investment versus promotional spending should be. However, there can be no debate as to whether the industry spends more on DTC advertising than on R&D, and any such claims are completely untrue.

PROS AND CONS OF DTC ADVERTISING

However, one might still question the need for any DTC advertising. Even if this amounts to only 1% of the industry's revenues, why not take this $4.8 billion and

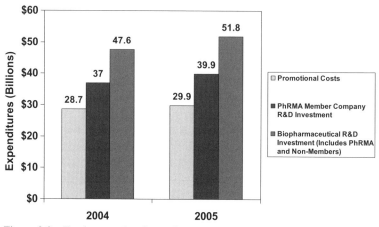

Figure 9.3   Total promotional spend as compared to R&D investment.

invest it in more R&D or maybe even roll back prescription drug prices by 1%? Indeed, DTC advertising is a controversial topic. The justification for it has always focused on patient education. DTC advertising is meant to provide patients with information about new medicines and treatments for diseases that previously were untreatable, such as fibromylagia as was described in Chapter 7. Furthermore, it is believed that patients would be encouraged by DTC advertising to open a dialogue with their doctor about medical conditions and illnesses—communication that might not have previously existed. Obviously, this dialogue can lead to the physician prescribing the advertised medication for the patient, as the *USA Today*/Kaiser/Harvard School of Public Health Survey shows. However, regardless of what prompts someone to visit a physician, this session provides an opportunity to discuss other treatment options such as better diet, more exercise, smoking cessation, and so on. Furthermore, another survey, "The 10th Annual National Survey on Consumer Reaction to DTC Pharmaceutical Advertising," showed that the most common action taken by a consumer in response to a DTC advertisement—before, during and after a prescription is filled—is more information seeking. This educational aspect is important in the overall management of health care because many people are not taking needed medicines. A study carried out by the RAND Corporation showed that Americans receive about half of the recommended preventative or acute care for chronic conditions such as high cholesterol, hypertension, or diabetes.[8] This study found that effective medications for these and other conditions are underutilized. The more patients know, the better off they can be.

There are, however, a variety of concerns about DTC advertising. One issue is whether DTC advertising causes the use of new, higher-cost drugs instead of cheaper generic alternatives. This doesn't appear to be the case because it has already been pointed out that physicians prescribe a different drug the majority of the time.[7] A second concern surrounded the patient–physician relationship in that an awkwardness could develop as a result of a patient demanding a drug that the physician thought was inappropriate for the situation. The FDA conducted a survey on this topic and, of 500 physicians polled, 91% believed that the patient did not try to influence the course of treatment in a manner that could have been harmful.[9] A final concern has been that a DTC advertisement could contain misleading information about the drug being promoted. It must be noted that the FDA has a separate unit— the Division of Drug Marketing, Advertising and Communications (DDMAC)—with the responsibility for reviewing prescription drug advertising to ensure that the information is neither misleading nor false.

In recognition of the fact that the industry is responsible for compliance with FDA regulations, PhRMA developed a set of guiding principles that are designed to conform to FDA requirements and assist companies in their efforts to comply with FDA legal requirements. These 15 principles are designed to ensure that DTC advertising provides accurate information, makes claims supported by scientific evidence, reflects the risk–benefit for the medicine, and is consistent with the label approved by the FDA.[10] In addition, in recognition of the fact that the risk–benefit profile of a new drug is not fully understood until a broader population is exposed to the drug, DTC advertising does not begin until the medicine has been on the market for a year.

One of these guiding principles is of particular interest.

13. In terms of content and placement, DTC television and print advertisements should be targeted to avoid audiences that are not age appropriate for the messages involved.

The principle was generated in part due to the concerns of having commercials for erectile dysfunction products on television during prime viewing hours. And perhaps that is the proverbial "elephant in the room" when it comes to DTC advertising. It is these commercials that are used by critics of DTC advertising as examples of all that is wrong with pharmaceutical industry practices. Few had ever heard of the term "erectile dysfunction" until a blue pill called Viagra arrived.

THE STORY OF VIAGRA®

Erectile dysfunction (ED), also known as impotence, was a condition that had been neglected by health care providers prior to 1998. There were a variety of reasons for this. First of all, ED was thought to be psychogenic in origin—that is, that the problem existed only in a subject's mind. Second, there were few treatments for ED; and those that did exist, such as penile implants or injection therapies, were incredibly unappealing. And yet, this is a highly prevalent condition and, as the longevity of the general population increases, the cases of ED continue to grow. For men aged 40–49, the prevalence of severe ED is 5% and for moderate ED it is 17%; for men aged 70–79, these rates are 15% and 34%, respectively.[11]

ED results not just from psychological factors but also from various biological conditions. These include diabetes, atherosclerosis (the same process that results in arterial plaques can also limit blood flow to the penis) and benign prostatic hyperplasia. In addition, smoking, alcohol, certain medications like antidepressants, and even prolonged bicycling (pressure from the bicycle seat can compress nerves and blood flow to the penis) can result in ED. When men visit a doctor to seek help for their ED, it is fairly common that their physical examination will uncover an underlying disease or condition causing their ED. DTC advertising for ED drugs, in fact, is believed to have resulted in thousands of patients being diagnosed with diabetes or cardiovascular disease. These commercials have caused men to seek new treatments and, for some, their overall health has benefited as a result.

The program that led to Viagra began in 1983, a time when little research was being done on drugs to treat ED. Dr. Simon Campbell, who at the time headed Medicinal Chemistry in Pfizer's R&D laboratories in Sandwich, England, believed that by inhibiting a particular enzyme, known as phosphodiesterase (PDE), one could initiate a cascade of biological events that culminates in vasodilatation and a reduction in blood pressure. So this program initially was envisioned to come up with a novel treatment for hypertension. The first hurdle to overcome was to determine which of the phosphodiesterases was the target to pursue because there had been about nine distinct PDEs known at the time. Biologist Frank Burslem and his colleagues worked hard over 12 months doing studies aimed at locating where the PDEs were present physiologically. They found PDE-5 to be an interesting enzyme because it was present in very high concentrations in vascular smooth muscles, suggesting that an inhibitor of PDE-5 could enhance blood flow. Interestingly, PDE-5 was not present in the kidney and so a PDE-5 inhibitor was unlikely to be a robust antihypertensive agent. However, it did appear that a PDE-5 inhibitor could be very effective in treating angina—a condition in which severe chest pain occurs as a result of the insufficient blood flow to the heart. Angina is a symptom of underlying heart disease, and it is thought that 7 million people suffer from this in the United States alone.

Thus, this program evolved into one looking for specific PDE-5 inhibitors for the treatment of angina. Chemist Nick Terrett and his colleagues identified an interesting series of compounds highlighted by one with the code name, UK-92,480, which was first synthesized in 1988. Preclinical studies were quite promising, and the compound moved on to clinical trials. The initial trials, however, were disappointing. UK-92,480 was safe and well-tolerated in volunteers, but there was minimal impact on important cardiovascular parameters such as blood pressure, heart rate, cardiac output, and blood flow. The compound was nearly discontinued, and this would have occurred had not an interesting observation been made. In one study that was done in 1992 in Wales, male volunteers who were taking 50 mg of UK-92,480 every 8 hours for 10 days reported more erections. It wasn't far-fetched that such activity could be caused by a PDE-5 inhibitor like UK-92,480. The same biological mechanisms that were hypothesized to help in treating angina could instead be coming into play in the penis, resulting in enhanced blood flow to this organ.

It must be noted that there was no mention of erections by the volunteers in the first studies of UK-92,480. Thus, there was a worry that this result was an aberration. In addition, in the only study where erections were seen, UK-92,480 was dosed twice a day for 2 days and so, even if this effect was real, the compound might not have a sufficiently rapid onset of action. There were other concerns as well. In the early 1990s, regulatory guidelines for a drug for ED were virtually nonexistent, as were diagnostic criteria and even instruments to measure efficacy. And if that weren't enough, it was unclear as to whether there would even be a market for such a drug. After all, in the early 1990s, this subject was still taboo.

Pfizer did some market research on this condition. As is often the case when the current treatments are unacceptable, the ED market was small and so a drug to treat ED might not generate much in the way of sales. There was also a belief, however, that the number of ED patients was understated since men were reluctant to tell their doctors they had this problem. Thus, maybe there would be a significant demand for such a drug. In the face of this uncertainty, Pfizer carried out a pilot study in men with ED, with 12 taking a single 50-mg dose and 12 receiving a placebo. The results proved to be very encouraging: 10 out of 12 on UK-92,480 reported improved erections, whereas only 2 of 12 on placebo reported any improvement. UK-92,480 was given the generic name of sildenafil and eventually sold under the trademark of Viagra.

It is important to note that Viagra doesn't induce erections on its own. It doesn't work without sexual stimulation, and this is probably why erections were not reported in the initial angina studies. It is likely that those patients in the Welsh study were thinking of sex and thereby prompted the discovery of one of the more famous medicines in history.

However, in 1994 this compound was still a long way from being a drug. The unprecedented mechanism of action of Viagra challenged the development team led by Dr. Ian Osterloh, who expressed this situation quite simply:

> No one had developed an oral drug for ED. There were no guidelines on how to do it. The team spent a long of time debating trial design, patient selection criteria, efficacy measures, and so on.

As happened with Zoloft for PTSD and Lyrica for fibromyalgia, the team worked with the FDA and other regulatory agencies to gain agreement on efficacy measures. Discussions focused on what criteria would be considered for meaningful efficacy. As part of this work, Pfizer helped to develop the "International Index of Erectile Function," which is the gold standard for evaluating ED.[12]

Viagra was tested in most forms of ED, such as severe organ disease caused by diabetes or spinal cord injuries as well as disease originating from mixed psychogenic/organic causes. The first major trial was begun in 1994 and involved 300 patients in Europe. The results were as good as could have been hoped for: using a 50-mg dose, 88% of patients using Viagra reported improved erections as compared to 39% on placebo. The drug was very well tolerated, with the most common side effects being headache and facial flushing. There are also visual effects: Viagra weakly inhibits the PDE-6 enzyme and thus can cause the patient to experience increased light sensitivity or a blue tint to their vision. However, this is a transient effect. Finally, Viagra cannot be used by men with cardiovascular problems that require treatment with nitroglycerin.

The NDA for Viagra was filed in 1997 and approved by the FDA on March 27, 1998. While it immediately became one of the most talked about medicines of all time, it also became a successful product as well, with sales exceeding

$1.7 billion in 2007. But because of its fame, people are generally surprised to hear that Viagra accounts for less than 4% of Pfizer's sales. But make no mistake about the impact this drug has had on patients with ED. Former Pfizer CEO Bill Steere once said that he received more heartfelt letters from Viagra users than from users of any other Pfizer product. An excerpt from one such letter is given below.

> Before I took part in the study I was heavily depressed. The feeling of being unable to have a normal sexual relationship with my wife was driving me insane. … I have no doubt that entering the study saved our family from much grief. It would not be exaggerating to say it probably saved my marriage and possibly my life.

A LIFE-EXTENDING USE FOR SILDENAFIL (VIAGRA®)

While Viagra is well known for its effectiveness in ED, its active ingredient, sildenafil, is also quite effective in treating another disease. Pulmonary arterial hypertension (PAH) is a condition in which the arteries of the lungs are constricted. This forces the heart to work hard to pump blood through the lungs. In time, the heart muscle weakens and loses its ability to pump enough blood throughout the body, thereby leading to heart failure. There are two types of PAH: primary PAH, a rare genetic disorder of which there are 300 new cases annually in the United States; and secondary PAH, in which the increased pressure of the lung's blood vessels results from other medical conditions. In either form of PAH, patients have limited capacity for physical activity and, as the heart grows weaker, energy wanes and patients become bedridden. Eventually, they develop heart failure, which leads to premature death.

Interestingly, PDE-5 is the main form of the phosphodiesterases found in the pulmonary vasculature. Given that Viagra was known to cause vasodilatation that led to enhanced blood flow in the penis where there is also a high concentration of PDE-5, physicians treating PAH patents began to experiment with Viagra to see if people with PAH could benefit by being treated with this PDE-5 inhibitor. In fact, the compound anecdotally appeared to be helpful in PAH patients. As a result, Pfizer sponsored clinical studies to explore the potential of the active ingredient of Viagra—sildenafil—for treating PAH.

The major endpoint in any clinical trial for PAH is a 6-minute walking distance test conducted on a treadmill. This test is an independent predictor of death in patients with PAH. The results of a major study of sildenafil in PAH are shown in Figure 9.4.[13] In this study, 278 PAH patients were randomly assigned to one of the following regimens: 20, 40, or 80 mg of sildenafil orally three times per day or placebo. All doses of sildenafil gave equally robust increases in treadmill walking distances after 12 weeks. Furthermore, 222 of these patients continued their sildenafil therapy for a year and they were able to maintain this improvement. Sildenafil improved exercise capacity, functional ability, and hemodynamics in these patients. On the basis of this pivotal study, the FDA approved the use of sildenafil for PAH patients to improve their exercise ability with a recommended dose of 20 mg given three times a day. To avoid confusion, this form of sildenafil is sold as Revatio and

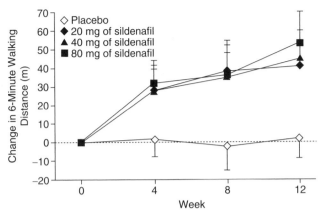

Figure 9.4   Increase in 6-minute walking distance with sildenafil as compared to placebo.

comes in little white pills to distinguish it from the more famous version sold as blue diamond-shaped pills.

Thus, a project started in 1985 to seek a new treatment for hypertension resulted in two products: one that treats a condition that was difficult to discuss and one to treat a condition that leads to heart failure. Certainly, none of this was envisioned more than two decades ago. But this is what often happens in pharmaceutical research. Scientists invent molecules to understand the causes and ultimately provide new treatments for diseases, and new treatments may be developed for diseases different from those initially intended.

The recent 10th anniversary of the approval and marketing of Viagra prompted a spate of stories in the media chronicling the history of this drug. Comics have gotten many a laugh from Viagra jokes, Viagra has been mentioned in movies and television shows, and it is a topic of conversation at cocktail parties, particularly around sex and aging. And all stories about Viagra also make mention of the TV advertisements from Bob Dole to "Viva Viagra." The FDA approval of Viagra occurred at about the same time the FDA allowed DTC advertising. This has caused discomfort for some. But for many, the ability to feel that ED was no longer a taboo subject has changed their lives. Viagra improves the quality of life, not just for the ED patient but also for their partner. As a result, the patient's self-esteem increases, as does their ability to maintain intimate relationships. For many, many people this is a very important medicine.

CHAPTER 10

INDUSTRY DOES NOT CARE ABOUT DISEASES OF THE DEVELOPING WORLD

Drug companies spend more on advertising and marketing than research, more on research on lifestyle drugs than on life saving drugs, and almost nothing on diseases that affect developing countries only.[1]

THIS QUOTE is a veritable trifecta of insults to the pharmaceutical industry. This author isn't someone in need of an attention grabbing headline. The author is Professor Joseph Stiglitz of Columbia University, who was the chief economist of the World Bank from 1997 to 2000 and who won the Nobel Prize for economics in 2001. I would hope that the previous chapter would address his first point. I would also hope that most would agree that drugs to treat cancer, AIDS, life-threatening bacterial infections, heart disease, arthritis, diabetes, and so on, are not lifestyle drugs. But what about Professor Stiglitz's last point? Pharmaceutical companies are not philanthropic organizations. They are profit-making entities that operate in an intensively competitive arena. Do these companies callously ignore the diseases that plague developing countries?

First of all, pharmaceutical companies are leaders when it comes to corporate philanthropy. An article in *The Chronicle of Philanthropy* showed that in 2006 the top four corporate donors of cash and products combined were Pfizer ($1.7 billion), Merck ($826 million), Johnson and Johnson ($545 million), and Bristol-Myers Squibb ($528 million).[2] These are significant contributions amounting to roughly 2% of overall sales for these companies. Fifth overall was Microsoft ($436 million). As will be seen later in this chapter, significant amounts of these contributions go toward alleviating the disease burden in the developing world and so the claim that pharmaceutical companies spend almost nothing on helping to treat diseases of the third world is far from true. However, this is not a problem that is localized in one region of the world and thus can be ignored. Everyone owns it. This problem is a complicated one entwined with poverty, hunger, education, and access. There are three main areas that need to be addressed by all including pharmaceutical companies, specifically:

Drug Truths: Dispelling the Myths About Pharma R&D, by John L. LaMattina
Copyright © 2009 John Wiley & Sons, Inc.

- Poverty and disease
- Access to medicines
- R&D regarding neglected diseases

POVERTY AND DISEASE

In 2000, the United Nations adopted the "Millennium Development Goals," which were designed to uphold the principles of human dignity, equality, and equity at the global level. The very first of these goals is to eradicate extreme poverty and hunger with the specific target being the reduction in the population of those suffering from extreme poverty by at least 50% by 2015. From a health standpoint, the importance of this in improving the health of the poor was eloquently shown by Flanagin and Winkler[3] in the *Journal of the American Medical Association*:

> Poverty is an inveterate consequence and cause of ill health. Without financial resources, people cannot pay for basic human needs: food, water, sanitation, and healthcare services. In addition, poor people often live in poor countries that have limited or deteriorating healthcare systems and not enough physicians, nurses, and other trained healthcare workers.

In an interview Dr. Jeffrey Sachs, an architect of the United Nations' Millennium Development Goals, gave an excellent example of such problems:

> Malaria is largely preventable by simple technologies such as insecticide-treated bed nets and treatable by first-line medicines. Yet, in many cases, the medicines don't get to the children in time and they die. The U.S. championed what's called social marketing of bed nets, meaning that the bed nets are sold at discounted prices. Although only a dollar or two, many people simply can't afford this.[4]

The infrastructure issues facing the developing world are indeed challenging. Yet, there are simple measures that can add great value. A recent study in resource-poor areas in rural India showed that education of these populations about already available services resulted in 30% more prenatal exams, 27% more tetanus vaccinations, and 25% more infant vaccinations.[5] Another study estimated that by improving child nutrition, providing clean water and sanitation, and supplying clean household fuels to all children younger than 5 years old, there would be an annual reduction of child deaths of 800,000 (24%) in South Asia and 1.47 million (31%) in sub-Saharan Africa.[6]

The pharmaceutical industry is contributing to a variety of educational initiatives to help this situation. GlaxoSmithKline (GSK) in 2001 created the GSK African Malaria Partnership to implement behavioral change programs to aid in the prevention of malaria in vulnerable communities.[7] The ACCESS project, supported by the Novartis Foundation, has been used in Tanzanian districts where malaria has high prevalence rates. This program has informed people about the disease, improved the diagnosis of malaria, and increased access to medicines.[8] Astra Zeneca has partnered with the Red Cross to fight tuberculosis (TB) in poor areas in Central Asia by increasing the awareness of the disease, encouraging people to seek early diagnosis when TB is suspected, improving treatment compliance, and providing ongoing care and support.[9] These are just a few examples of key education initiatives that are aimed at reducing the incidence of these disease in the developing world.

ACCESS TO MEDICINES

While education initiatives, improvements in sanitation, and having sufficient number of health care providers are all critical in reducing the burden of disease in the developing world, there is no doubt that having access to life-saving medicines is key to success. Almost every major pharmaceutical company has programs designed to provide free medicines to such people in need. Bayer has provided to the World Health Organization (WHO) over 2.5 million tablets of Lampit to fight Chagas disease (a common form of sleeping sickness in South America).[10] Sanofi-aventis has also worked with the WHO to reduce African typanosomiasis (another form of sleeping sickness) by providing over one million injectable doses of the combination of pentamidine/melarsorprol/effornithine along with $25 million to support its distribution. In 2007, Merck donated $125 million worth of medicines and vaccines to fight a variety of diseases in the third world.[11] Pfizer's Diflucan partnership program has provided over $500 million worth of this important medication to treat fungal infections associated with HIV/AIDS to governments and non-governmental organizations for free in more than 80 eligible countries in need.[12]

However, many industry critics feel that such programs are not nearly enough and that many more medications should be given away to countries in need. A number of countries are going even further by pursuing "compulsory licenses," which are devices used by governments to circumvent IP rights in an attempt to make patented medicines more accessible. This basically is a method to ignore patents. They are used by governments to manufacture and sell patented medicines, without regard to intellectual property rights or compensation to the inventors. Under World Trade Organization rules, governments can break a patent in cases of national emergency or when attempts to obtain permission from the patent holder on "reasonable" commercial terms have failed. Thailand has already used this tactic for two patented drugs for HIV/AIDS, efavirenz and lopinavir/retonavir, as well as for an anticoagulant to treat heart disease. This is occurring despite the fact that Thailand receives steep discounts on these drugs to begin with. However, Thailand's government feels that they should pay the same for medicines as do countries in sub-Saharan Africa, even though Thailand is far better off economically. There are a number of issues with the compulsory license scheme. Table 10.1 compares the leading causes of death in the world as divided by low/middle-income countries and high-income countries.[13] When one usually thinks about developing world mortality, diseases like HIV/AIDS, malaria, TB, and rare infectious diseases come to mind. However, the leading causes of death in these countries are heart attacks, strokes, and pneumonia—very similar to deaths in higher income countries. Theoretically, a country could declare compulsory licenses basically on the entire gamut of the

TABLE 10.1   Leading Causes of Death in the World by Income Group, 2001

Low- and Middle-Income Countries			High-Income Countries		
Cause	Deaths (millions)	Percentage of Total Deaths	Cause	Deaths (millions)	Percentage of Total Deaths
Ischemic heart disease	5.70	11.8	Ischemic heart disease	1.36	17.3
Cerebrovascular disease	4.61	9.5	Cerebrovascular disease	0.78	9.9
Lower respiratory infections	3.41	7.0	Trachea, bronchus, and lung cancers	0.46	5.8
HIV/AIDS	2.55	5.3	Lower respiratory infections	0.34	4.4
Perinatal conditions	2.49	5.1	Chronic obstructive pulmonary disease	0.30	3.8
Chronic obstructive pulmonary disease	2.38	4.9	Colon and rectal cancers	0.26	3.3
Diarrheal diseases	1.78	3.7	Alzheimer's disease/dementias	0.21	2.6
Tuberculosis	1.59	3.3	Diabetes mellitus	0.20	2.6
Malaria	1.21	2.5	Breast cancer	0.16	2.0
Traffic accidents	1.07	2.2	Stomach cancer	0.15	1.0

pharmaceutical industry's pipeline since the major causes of deaths in these countries are not solely due to tropical diseases. It might be argued that all people deserve the right to life-saving medicines and that big pharmaceuticals are so well off that they should simply permit this. These same life-saving medicines, however, have been generated by companies that must return a profit on their R&D investments in order to keep producing tomorrow's medical miracles. Furthermore, if compulsory licenses are to become the norm, it is difficult to believe that pharmaceutical companies would continue to invest any R&D in diseases that predominate in the developing world.

The pharmaceutical industry is cognizant of the economic issues that these countries face, and it has developed programs to improve access without compromising essential IP rights. For example, many drugs are sold on a "tiered" or "differential" pricing basis. This system is designed to make important medicines available in resource constrained countries at prices far below those charged in high income countries. The reason for this is obvious. Companies, while trying to maintain profitability, also recognize their responsibility to world health.

R&D IN NEGLECTED DISEASES

Despite the threats of compulsory licenses, the pharmaceutical industry continues to invest R&D funds in diseases not prevalent in high-income countries. Again, looking at Table 10.1, AIDS, diarrheal diseases, TB, and malaria account for 15% of deaths in poorer nations, yet these diseases are not on the top 10 list of the causes of death in wealthier countries. Despite this fact and despite the challenges presented by their current business environment, pharmaceutical companies nevertheless continue to do their part in alleviating the global burden of diseases. Astra Zeneca in 2003 established a research institute in Bangalore, India to find new treatments for TB. GSK has a dedicated drug discovery unit in Spain devoted to looking for drugs to treat malaria and TB. The Novartis Institute for Tropical Diseases has been established in Singapore and is focused on seeking new medicines for malaria and Dengue fever. And even in the face of potential compulsory licensing, a number of companies have maintained their R&D efforts in HIV/AIDS including Abbott, Boehringer-Ingelheim, Bristol-Myers Squibb, Pfizer and Schering-Plough.

And the industry contributes in even more ways. A large number of public–private partnerships exist such as the WHO's Special Program for Research and Training in Tropical Diseases. The role of industry in these collaborations includes the following:

1. Providing research expertise and resources for target identification and high-throughput screening

2. Advising on clinical trial design

3. Aiding in dossier preparation

4. Sharing manufacturing skills and formulation development

5. Providing medical training

In some ways the sharing of this expertise is at least as important as the donations of money and medicine. The teaching and mentoring that occurs in these relationships has a multiplying effect on the amount of R&D achievable for these diseases.

At times a single company can make an enormous contribution in the eradication of some of these diseases. A wonderful example is the work that Merck has done in attacking onchocerciasis, commonly known as river blindness. This disease is spread through black fly bites and is characterized by intense itching, disfiguring dermatitis, and eye lesions that eventually lead to blindness. Mectizan® (generic name: ivermectin) is a Merck drug that both relieves the itching and also halts progression of the disease towards blindness. What is also important is that Mectizan only needs to be dosed once annually. In 1987, Merck announced the formation of a partnership with the WHO, the World Bank, UNICEF, and various ministries of health, with the goal of eradicating river blindness—the second leading cause of preventable blindness. For their part, Merck agreed to donate Mectizan to all who needed it for as long as necessary.[14]

The results from this program have been remarkable. More than 69 million Mectizan treatments are being given annually across 33 different countries in Africa and Latin America. The WHO estimates that 40,000 cases of blindness are being prevented annually as a result of this. The value of the Mectizan donation in 2007 alone was $480 million. Furthermore, Mectizan has been found to be effective in treating lymphatic filariasis, another parasitic infection that is commonly referred to as elephantiasis because of the swelling it produces in arms and legs. This disease coexists with river blindness, and Merck has included free drug for this as well as for part of the Mectizan Donation Program. Former U.S. President Jimmy Carter has said that this program is one of the most remarkable, exciting, and inspiring partnerships that he's ever witnessed.

While river blindness is the second leading cause of preventable blindness, the leading cause is trachoma. Although trachoma is nonexistent in the developed world, it is endemic to developing countries. It is caused by a bacterium, *Chlamydia trachomatis*, and is spread through secretions from the eye, nose, and throat. Trachoma is prevalent in areas of poverty and poor hygiene resulting from lack of clean water. Trachoma causes the inside of the eyelid to scar badly, resulting in eyelashes turning inward; this leads to corneal scarring and then blindness. There is an initiative underway to eradicate trachoma, but before getting to that, a discussion of the discovery of an important antibacterial agent, Zithromax, is in order.

THE HISTORY OF ZITHROMAX®

Erythromycin is an important antibiotic that was discovered by scientists at Eli Lilly in the early 1950s. At the time, erythromycin represented a major breakthrough as it was superior to penicillin in treating certain types of infections and was able to be used in people who were allergic to penicillin. But erythromycin, even before the development of bacterial resistance to it, was limited in its clinical usefulness because it was ineffective against certain organisms such as *Haemophilus influenzae*, the cause of ear infections in children, and because its absorption from the gastrointestinal tract was erratic due to its instability in the gut. Despite these limitations, erythromycin was very useful in treating various streptococcus, staphylococcus, and chlamydia infections.

Pfizer had begun a program looking for the next-generation erythromycin in the 1970s. Chemists made a variety of modifications to the erythromycin molecule which would look promising in test tubes and in animal models, but which would fall short in humans. After 8 years, Pfizer management was ready to terminate the program. A lot of resources had been invested in this search, and the management felt that it was time to look into other opportunities. In fact, a last review of the program was scheduled for May 1982, a meeting that the scientific team felt would be the funeral for the project.

Earlier in 1982, Pfizer scientists had learned of a new type of erythromycin analog known as an azalide, which was discovered by Dr. Slobodan Djokie and his team at Pliva Pharmaceuticals in Eastern Europe. Pfizer chemists made a few azalides but, while they were active against a number of important bacteria in test tubes, these compounds lacked activity in animal models. The program began to wind down. Dr. Michael Bright, a chemist on the project, had a few more ideas to try. As luck would have it, on May 10, 1982, just a week before the scheduled funeral, the *in vitro* results for a compound, code named CP-62,993, became available and this compound proved to be more potent than anything the team had ever seen.[15] Mike and his colleagues quickly made more of CP-62,993 to test in animal models. The results were available on the morning of the big meeting. Mike's memory of that day is quite revealing.

> By the morning of the meeting—this wake where they planned to eulogize the program—the oral data had come back and it was great! So all morning we're Xeroxing the slides and putting our data together. We didn't even have time to tell the senior managers before getting to the meeting. I happened to be sitting in the back row. At the start of the meeting I literally had to step over people to get to Dr. John Niblack, who was in charge of Research then. I threw the data in front of him and said: "John, you have to look at this right now." He took one look at the data and asked: "Isn't this the most exciting thing we've ever seen?" Everyone agreed that this compound was what we had been looking for all these years. And the bottom line was that the program *didn't* end.

CP-62,993, generically known as azithromycin, was on its way. This azalide had unique properties that helped give it enhanced potency. Pfizer biologists found that azithromycin had much higher tissue levels than erythromycin.[16] This was important because this characteristic would allow the drug to get to localized sites of infection like abscesses or infections of the middle ear, liver, and lung. Further studies with azithromycin showed that it was readily taken up by phagocytes.[17] The term phagocyte means "cell eater" in Greek and is an appropriate name for a cell that digests intracellular bacteria. It is believed that azithromycin is fortuitously taken up by phagocytes and delivered directly to the site of infection. Azithromycin-loaded cells then act in concert with the phagocyte's bacteria killing mechanisms to eradicate these microbes. Thus, azithromycin turned out to be a wonderful antibiotic: it gets to difficult to reach infections and complements one's own immune system to knock out the infection. These properties also enable the drug to be dosed only once a day for 3 days, making compliance much easier.

The team was now off and running. The clinical plans were developed, centers to run the clinical trials were established, and patients were recruited. However, the team received a major jolt when the company sought a U.S. patent on azithromycin. They learned that Pliva had filed for a patent on azithromycin a month earlier. It turned out that Dr. Djokie had synthesized azithromycin in late 1981. Pfizer therefore rescinded its patent application and became a business partner with Pliva. This joint development program resulted in the drug's approval by the FDA in 1992, and it was given the brand name of Zithromax.[18] In recognition of the importance of this medicine, the American Chemical Society bestowed their "Heroes of Chemistry" award in 2000 to Slobodan Djokie, Gabriela Kobiehel, Mike Bright, and Art Girard, whose work, while carried out in separate companies and continents, led to a major new treatment for infectious diseases.

ZITHROMAX® FOR TRACHOMA AND MALARIA

Zithromax is especially effective against *Chlamydia trachomatis*, the bacterium responsible for causing trachoma. In 1998, Pfizer and the Edna McConnell Clark Foundation co-founded the International Trachoma Initiative (ITI). This public–

private partnership is dedicated to eliminating trachoma through health work or training, patient education, and Pfizer's donation of Zithromax. The ITI has provided 54 million treatments of Zithromax to trachoma patients in 15 countries as part of the WHO SAFE strategy (*S*urgery, *A*ntibiotics, *F*ace-washing, and *E*nvironmental improvement).[19] Over the last 10 years, the program has supported the training of thousands of health care workers around the world who, in turn, have completed more than 277,000 surgeries to treat advanced cases of trachoma. The results to date have been extremely encouraging. The SAFE strategy has been so successful in Morocco that trachoma has been eliminated in this country. Progress has been made in other locales as well. A recent report in the *New England Journal of Medicine* has documented that a single mass treatment of Zithromax in a Tanzanian village caused a remarkable drop in trachoma, and a second mass treatment resulted in the complete elimination of this organism 5 years later.[20] Because of such results, Dr. Joseph Cook, a professor of epidemiology at the University of North Carolina, has recently said:

> The early results achieved with the use of the SAFE strategy and azithromycin (Zithromax) mass treatment suggest that elimination of blinding trachoma by 2020 is entirely possible.[19]

Pfizer also has a major commitment in the development of a potential malaria treatment based on the combination of Zithromax dosed in combination with chloroquine. Zithromax alone does not provide sufficient efficacy in treating this disease. But the drug combination is particularly efficacious in eradicating this pathogen in patients as proven in two Phase 3 studies carried out in sub-Saharan Africa.[21a,b] The combination thus far appears well-tolerated, which is particularly important because this simple oral combination is attractive for the prevention of disease in pregnant women and children. Confirmatory trials in these populations are ongoing.

There is absolutely no financial benefit to Pfizer in carrying out studies of Zithromax/chloroquine in malaria. The same can be said for all of the studies and initiatives being carried out by other companies as has already been described. In fact, the altruistic work described here is only a small percentage of the work being done by the pharmaceutical industry in helping those suffering in the developing world. The International Federation of Pharmaceutical Manufacturers and Associations has a comprehensive description of what the industry is doing on their website.[22] Can the industry do more? Perhaps, but can't the same be said for all industries able to provide food, clean water, shelter, and roads to those less fortunate? As was stated at the beginning of this chapter, pharmaceutical companies are not philanthropic organizations; furthermore, these companies are in the midst of severe business challenges. Given this perspective, the amount of effort this industry is putting into treating even diseases of the developing world is noteworthy. To say that the industry spends almost nothing on diseases that affect developing countries is plainly wrong.

PART *IV*

THE FUTURE

T HE STORIES appear each January as an annual rite. They report on the FDA's annual summary of new drugs approved in the previous year with headlines like: "Where have all the new drugs gone: Industry's medicine cabinet running empty on compounds."[1] The stories quote Wall Street's pharmaceutical analysts, who hypothesize on the cause: major products losing patent protection, higher hurdles being set for new medicines in terms of safety and efficacy, and so on. The implication is that the pharmaceutical industry has lost its way, that its business model is broken, and that its current funk is not temporal.

These are paradoxical times. One might assume a "golden era" of new drug productivity. The unraveling of the human genome has provided a wealth of new information about the mechanisms underlying the causes of many new diseases. This explosion of information has, in turn, opened up a number of new targets for scientists pursuing new treatments for unmet medical needs. In this time of biological plenty, however, the pharmaceutical industry is struggling with mergers, cutbacks in R&D spending, and layoffs across the board. This is unfortunate because, as has been explained throughout this book, this industry is the primary source of new medicines and new treatments are needed for a host of diseases including cancer, Alzheimer's disease, diabetes, and so on. If the pharmaceutical industry is indeed broken, who else will capitalize on the opportunities being provided by recent scientific breakthroughs? A long-term decrease in the output of new medicines by the pharmaceutical industry would threaten the world's well-being.

CHAPTER 11

BIG PHARMA'S DAY HAS PASSED

MOST ARTICLES that discuss the declining productivity of the pharmaceutical industry point to data such as that shown in Figure 11.1 to describe the decline. This graph depicts the annual FDA approvals of new medical entities since 1996; indeed, this decrease is striking, particularly in comparison to 1996. It should be pointed out, however, that 1996 is a year that truly stands out. Far more drugs were approved that year than anytime before or since. There are a number of reasons why, but a major cause was the impact of the Prescription Drug User Fee Act (PDUFA) of 1992. Few remember that back in the late 1980s and early 1990s there was a "drug lag" in the U.S. versus other parts of the world. Because of a lack of resources at the FDA, drugs were approved at a much slower rate in the United States than in Europe. More than half of all drugs approved in the United States had been approved in Europe more than a year earlier.[1] Patients, advocacy groups, pharmaceutical companies, and physicians were all concerned that new important medications were being denied to Americans.

To solve this problem, Congress enacted PDUFA—a mechanism whereby charges were levied on pharmaceutical companies for each new drug application filed. The revenues from these "user fees" were used to hire 600 new drug reviewers and support staff. These new medical officers, chemists, pharmacologists, and other experts were tasked with clearing the backlog of new drug applications (NDAs) awaiting approval. They would reduce review times of NDAs to 12 months for standard applications and to 6 months for priority applications that involved significant advances over existing treatments. In 1995, the user fee for a full NDA was $208,000. This fee has grown substantially over the years and is now $1,178,000.[2] PDUFA proved highly successful. As a result of the growth of the FDA, the backlog of the 1990s was indeed eliminated, review times were brought in line with other parts of the world, and new drugs were made available sooner. And the record number of NDAs approved in 1996, in part, demonstrates this impact.

To get a true sense of trends in the productivity of the pharmaceutical industry, it is helpful to look at NDA approvals across a broader time period than just the last decade. A recent publication has done just that.[3] Schmid and Smith examined NDA approvals in the United States in 10-year increments starting in 1945. Their findings surprised many. As can be seen in Figure 11.2, there has been a steady growth in drug approvals since the 1940s, with one exception—the 1965–1974 period—and there is an important event that occurred in this latter period that helps to explain

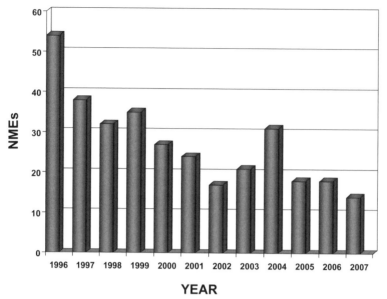

Figure 11.1   FDA approvals of new medical entities: 1996–2007.

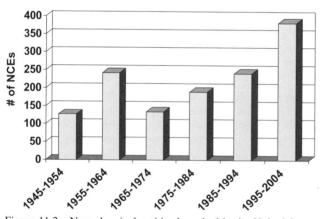

Figure 11.2   New chemical entities launched in the United States, 1945–2004.

the 1965–1974 decline. In the late 1950s, a drug called thalidomide was marketed in Europe; this agent was prescribed to pregnant women to help overcome morning sickness and to help them sleep. Unfortunately, insufficient toxicology testing had been done on this drug before it was approved. Thalidomide is a teratogen, a compound that interferes with the growth of the fetus and causes severe birth defects. Thousands of babies were born with severe deformities because their mothers took this drug. Fortunately, thalidomide was never approved by the FDA. However, because of the public alarm and outcry that justifiably arose from this horror, the

Kefauver–Harris Drug Act was established in 1962. This legislation completely overhauled the drug approval process, revamping the methods and procedures used by pharmaceutical companies to get drugs developed and approved. Figure 11.2 shows that it took over a decade for pharmaceutical industry productivity to rebound, but clearly better, safer drugs resulted from this event. This example shows how external events and changing requirements for drug approval can have a profound impact on overall productivity. Given that the drug discovery and development process is 12–15 years in length, it takes time to adapt to major changes to the drug review process.

Thalidomide demonstrates another surprising facet of drug development.[4] In the 1960s Jacob Sheskin, while working at Hadassah Hospital at Hebrew University in Jerusalem, was trying to help one of his leprosy patients sleep. He found some thalidomide and, remembering that it had helped patients with psychological problems sleep, he tried it on one of his patents. Surprisingly, the response to thalidomide in this patient and others was dramatic. Within days, most of the symptoms of leprosy disappeared. In what is a great example of the appropriate use of a drug once its risk–benefit is understood, thalidomide has become the drug of choice to treat leprosy, albeit under conditions carefully controlled by physicians. Furthermore, collaborative work done in the 1990s to elucidate thalidomide's mode of action led to its approval for the treatment of multiple myeloma, a form of cancer. This would have been unthinkable in 1962.

Although Figure 11.2 shows that productivity has increased in the ensuing decades, what about the quality of the compounds being produced? Has innovation also kept pace? Schmid and Smith also looked at this point as well. They used the FDA's own designation of "priority reviews" as an indication of innovation, and they looked at these trends over the past 60 years. As shown in Figure 11.3, while the numbers vary a great deal from year to year, overall there appears to be an upward trend in innovation over this timeframe.

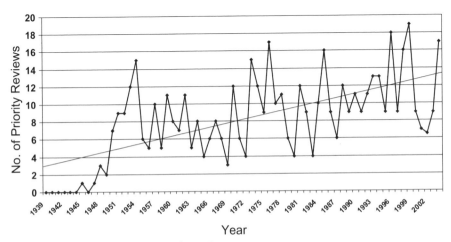

Figure 11.3   Number of FDA priority reviews per year.

Despite the increase in quality and output from the pharmaceutical industry over the past decades, it is unlikely that the Schmid–Smith total in 1995–2004 will be exceeded in 2005–2014, especially since less than 60 approvals have been registered in the 2005–2007 timeframe. While there are a variety of reasons for this decline, there are in my view three major factors:

1. Industry consolidation
2. Increased studies needed in NDAs to demonstrate drug safety
3. Increased studies needed in NDAs for drug differentiation

As was discussed in Chapter 6, the pharmaceutical industry has undergone dramatic consolidation over the past 10 years. Consolidations make great business sense as a way to remove duplication, reduce costs, and produce synergies. Experience to date shows that all of this does occur. However, these mergers drive cost reductions across all parts of these companies, including R&D. Major consolidations can result in fewer overall scientists in R&D and fewer research sites at these companies. An examination of the "family tree" for some companies is quite revealing. Sanofi-aventis has its roots in the following companies (some also resulting from mergers!): Marion Merrill Dow, Roussel-Uclaf, Hoescht, Rorer, Rhone-Poulenc, Fisons, Synthelabo, and Sanofi. Pfizer can be traced back through many companies including Warner-Lambert, Parke-Davis, Upjohn, Searle, Pharmacia, Jouvenal, Farmitalia, and Monsanto (pharmaceutical unit), as well as biotech companies such as Agouron, SUGEN and Vicuron. As part of these consolidations, Pfizer closed major research labs around the globe in Skokie, Illinois; Kalamazoo, Michigan; Ann Arbor, Michigan; Nagoya, Japan; and Amboise and Fresnes, France. Similar closures have occurred as a result of other mergers as well. While specific numbers are difficult to obtain across the industry, in this era of consolidation, it is unlikely that there has been any growth in big Pharma in terms of scientists producing new medicines and it is likely that there has been a decrease. This deficit has been made up in part by the emergence of the biotech industry, but overall there are fewer competitors in this space and this is likely having an impact on the invention and development of new drugs.

In addition, mergers cause disruptions and delays. When mergers occur, drug pipelines need to be consolidated and weaker programs eliminated. In many cases, early projects are moved to new locations; in some cases, entire therapeutic area teams can be shifted across continents. It is also common to introduce new business models that improve utilization of resources such as centralizing toxicology research in one location or concentrating drug formulation work in another. All of these changes make great business sense and, in the long run, increase efficiency. But they take time to implement. It is difficult to measure the overall impact on productivity that occurs as a result of reorganizations like these. A Nobel Laureate once told me that it can take three years to move a highly respected academic researcher from one university to another and restore his or her lab to full productivity. The pharmaceutical industry is less patient, but it is safe to assume that major mergers can result in 12-month delays in programs for which scientists and resources are translocated.

The second reason for the slowdown in NDA filings is the demand for more safety data in every drug's dossier. Any R&D head can describe examples showing how much bigger NDAs are now as compared to the filings of just a decade ago. As was discussed in Chapter 8, the amount of data included in the Celebrex NDA dwarfed that of any previous NSAID NDA. Overall, this is a very good thing for regulators, physicians, payers, and patients. Experimental medicines are now being tested in more patients and for longer periods of time than ever before. As a result, more is known about the safety of a new medicine when it is launched. These additional and longer studies do come at a price: they add both time and cost to programs. Dr. Janet Woodcock, Director of the FDA's Center for Drug Evaluation and Research, acknowledged this in an interview with Reuters in May 2008.[5] Pharmaceutical companies have adjusted, but the impact in NDA filings has been felt over the past 5 years. Presumably, Phase 3 programs underway across the industry are more comprehensive as a result of these higher expectations and so, in a sense, are bottled up.

Beyond showing that the risk–benefit profile for a new medicine is highly favorable, another *key* hurdle has grown dramatically since the turn of the century. What value does the new medicine bring over existing therapies? Until recently, differentiating studies could be done in Phase 4 after a new medicine was on the market. That is no longer true. Differentiation studies are now being done upfront so that they can be included in the initial NDA filing. In fact, if these differentiations do not show an advantage over existing therapies, the company will likely choose not to file the NDA at all. An excellent example of this was described in Chapter 3 in the discussion of the Phase 3 program for torcetrapib. This program included 38 clinical studies involving 25,000 patients, some treated for as long as 5 years, and was designed to show that the combination of torcetrapib with Lipitor would be superior to Lipitor alone. As you now know, the results showed that this was not the case. But it was critical to show that this new drug was superior to existing therapy to justify approval of its NDA. Not every new medicine will require this degree of differentiation. But, a decade ago, no such studies would have been carried out prior to a drug's approval. These studies add to the complexity and cost of clinical trials and have lengthened NDA filings. And much like the impact of expanded safety and toleration studies, these factors have also been built into the late-stage clinical programs across the industry.

It is my view that the following three changes to the pharmaceutical industry landscape—consolidation, increased safety studies, and increased differentiation studies—have had as big an impact on NDA filings as the Kefauver–Harris Drug Act of 1962. Thus, if one were to predict how the 2005–2014 NDA approvals will compare to the previous decades, there will likely be a decrease as compared to 1995–2004. However, there are signs that this decline is temporary. The pharmaceutical industry has adapted to these environmental changes and, as occurred in the 1960s, productivity will again rise.

There is growing evidence that supports this optimism. In 2006, the Tufts Center for the Study of Drug Development reported that the rate at which new drugs entered clinical testing increased by 52% in the 2003–2005 period as compared to 1998–2002.[6] This report also pointed out that the number of drugs that

	PHASE 1	PHASE 2	PHASE 3
MERCK			
December 2002	4	5	7
December 2007	25	15	7
PFIZER			
August 2002	22	21	6
August 2007	38	47	11

Figure 11.4   Growth of pipelines at Merck and Pfizer.

entered clinical trials had *declined* 21% from 1993–1997 to 1998–2002. The fact that pipelines were declining in 1998–2002 proved to be a predictor of fewer NDA filings that is now being seen. Similarly, the pipeline growth seen in 2003–2005 should also be predictive of more compounds emerging into the marketplace.

One can look at pharmaceutical company websites and also follow pipeline growth. In their quest to provide greater transparency to investors and the medical community, many pharmaceutical companies are posting their development pipelines on their websites. These pipelines are typically updated twice a year, thereby allowing people to measure a company's R&D progress over a period of time. Across the board, pharmaceutical pipelines are growing and Figure 11.4 lists two specific examples: Merck and Pfizer.[7]

Having a bigger pipeline does not necessarily guarantee more NDAs; these compounds must still overcome all the hurdles previously outlined in terms of efficacy, safety, and differentiation. Nevertheless, with many of the major pharmaceutical companies developing the largest pipelines in memory and with the maturing of biotech company portfolios with more late-stage development candidates, it is hard to believe that there won't be a resurgence of new drug approvals across multiple therapeutic areas in the coming years which will greatly benefit patients around the world. Nowhere is this more evident than in the tremendous advances being made in new drugs to treat cancer.

NEW CANCER DRUGS

In his State of the Union address in 1971, President Richard M. Nixon described his "War on Cancer," asking the nation for the levels of effort focused on the Manhattan Project or the Apollo Lunar Mission. On December 23, 1971, he signed the National Cancer Act into law which committed an additional $100 million to be added to the National Cancer Institute (NCI) for cancer research. Yet, unlike the successful landing of a man on the moon, there was no quick success. More than three decades after Nixon's proclamation, this war is still being fought. Some people claim that the War on Cancer failed. Such criticism, however, stems from a lack of understanding of the difficulties in curing this disease. Dr. Vincent DeVita, who was the director of the NCI, has correctly pointed out that approximately $50 billion has been spent on cancer research since 1971 and 80% of this has gone into just understanding the root causes of this disease.[8] Until recently, cancer was treated with cytotoxic drugs, chemotherapeutic agents that kill fast-dividing cancer cells. Unfortunately, these agents can also damage normal cells, and this relative lack of selectivity results in the severe side affects associated with cancer chemotherapy.

The basic research funded by the War on Cancer increased the understanding of cancer molecular biology such that mechanisms specific to tumor growth were elucidated. Research showed that cancer was not a single disease but rather a broad set of diseases resulting from aberrant cell growth caused by mutations in a variety of biological pathways. These triggers for aberrant cell growth are called oncogenes, genes which when activated turn normal cells into tumor cells. The basic research funded by the War on Cancer provided drug hunters just what they needed, namely, potential targets for novel drugs that, if effective, could specifically destroy tumor cells while causing little, if any, damage to normal cells. In essence, these potential drugs could be more effective in treating cancer than older cytotoxics and could prove safer as well.

Companies both large and small began to invest heavily into cancer research in the 1990s; as a result, there has been an explosion in potential new medicines for cancer pipelines across the industry unlike anything ever seen. We now envisage a time when cancer becomes a disease controlled by medicines, rather than a death sentence. It is possible that in the future a cancer patient will be treated with a "cocktail" of agents, not unlike the current HIV/AIDS treatment. These agents might (1) starve tumors in a patient by preventing them from growing blood vessels, thereby blocking the tumors from getting nutrients (a process called anti-angiogenesis); (2) reawaken the immune system to help fight the cancer; and (3) block the biological cascade that is allowing the tumor to proliferate. Progress being made in each of these areas is outlined below.

The person who first proposed that cancer could be treated by preventing angiogenesis was the late Dr. Judah Folkman. He believed that this approach would cause tumors to wither and die.[9] Initially, others were skeptical. But in the 1980s, a protein known as vascular endothelial growth factor (VEGF) was discovered and found to be a regulator of blood vessel growth. In the 1990s, scientists at Genentech developed an antibody that targets the receptor that binds VEGF. By blocking this receptor, they predicted that VEGF would be ineffective in helping a tumor grow needed blood vessels. In fact, this antibody proved to be extremely efficacious first in animal studies and then in the clinic.[10] In 2004, Genentech received FDA approval for this agent sold as Avastin® (generic name: bevacizumab) for the treatment of colon cancer in combination with 5-fluorouracil. It has since also been approved to be used in combination with other agents for lung cancer. Thus, more than 30 years after Folkman's hypothesis that an agent that blocks tumors from growing blood vessels would be an effective cancer treatment, his vision was recognized with a totally new treatment modality. It is obviously frustrating to patients that the process from idea to new medicines can take so long, but this is the reality of the drug discovery–development–approval process.

There is no doubt that Avastin has become a valuable anticancer agent. But as has been described in previous chapters, scientists seek to improve upon break-through therapies. Given the complexity of cancer, researchers sought compounds that combined anti-angiogenesis activity with other activities that inhibit internal growth drivers of a tumor with the hypothesis being that inhibiting multiple growth factors simultaneously would result in broader antitumor activities. Scientists at SUGEN[11] did just that. They discovered Sutent (generic name: sunitinib), a compound that blocks receptors involved in angiogenesis (VEGFs and PDGFβ) but also blocks other receptors, such as KIT and FLT3, known to play a role in driving the growth of certain tumors.[12] This compound has proven to be remarkable in treating different forms of cancer. It was approved by the FDA in 2006 for two indications: first, in advanced renal cell carcinoma (the most common form of kidney cancer) where Sutent provided significantly longer progression-free survival and with a much higher response rate than the standard therapy, Interferon Alfa®[13]; second, in advanced gastrointestinal stromal tumors resistant to Gleevec® for which there was no treatment.[14]

Even more noteworthy are early Phase 2 studies with Sutent including one in patients with breast cancer who had failed prior treatment with standard agents. These studies showed that a number of patients who had already received other treatments responded to single agent Sutent, albeit with an overall response rate of about 11%. Figure 11.5 is a scan of one Phase 2 patient that shows significant tumor shrinkage after just two cycles of therapy. (The tumor is highlighted in the circle.) These results are representative of one patient and are not seen universally, but this result bodes well for the potential of Sutent in this devastating disease. Sutent is now in Phase 3 studies for breast cancer as well as for lung and colon cancer.

A second novel approach to combating cancer involves activating a patient's immune system to help fight the cancer, an area of research familiarly referred to as immunotherapy. As tumors grow and spread, the immune system is inhibited such that the abnormal antigens on tumor cells are no longer recognized and so the immune system spares the tumor cells. Essentially, a "brake" is put on the immune system. This is known as immune tolerance. Scientists are exploring a number of

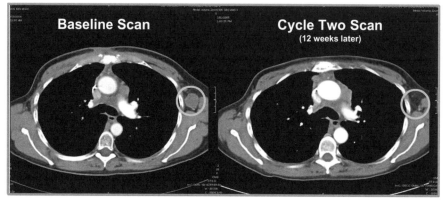

Figure 11.5   Activity of Sutent in a breast cancer patient who had failed with standard therapies.

ways to resolve immune tolerance, one of which involves blocking the actions of a protein known as cytotoxic T-lymphocyte antigen 4 (CTLA-4). When CTLA-4 binds to T cells, which are important to the function of the immune system, they are inactivated. Scientists felt that if they could prevent this action of CTLA-4, the T cells would be reactivated and the "brake" released so that the immune system would recognize the tumor cells as foreign. In order to achieve this, companies have sought antibodies to the receptor where CTLA-4 binds. Two such antibodies, tremelimumab and ipilimumab, are in Phase 3 studies. Tremelimumab has been studied as a single agent in metastatic melanoma, a serious form of skin cancer. Initial results with this antibody had proven quite promising. Figure 11.6 details a patient's progress from February 2005 to May 2006 on tremelimumab. After being given monthly doses of this drug, the disease was amazingly eradicated after 15 months. Furthermore, biopsies taken during the treatment showed the presence of dense infiltrates of immune cells specific against the tumor, providing evidence to support the concept that tremelimumab was in fact acting by an immune-mediated process.

Despite these early results, the drug failed to show superiority to standard chemotherapy already used to treat this disease. As a result, Pfizer has stopped the clinical studies on tremelimumab as a single agent treatment for metastatic melanoma. The reason for this is not yet understood. Pfizer still continues to study tremelimumab in combination with other agents to treat cancers such as colorectal cancer and non-small-cell lung cancer. Optimism remains that immunotherapy will be an excellent complement to anti-angiogenesis agents and agents that block

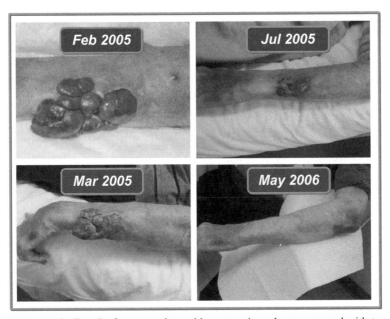

Figure 11.6   Results for one patient with metastatic melanoma treated with tremelimumab. See color insert.

tumor cell growth. Furthermore, Bristol-Myers Squibb and Medarex, the developers of ipilimumab are continuing their Phase 3 program with this agent. While tremelimumab and ipilimumab share a common mechanism of action, they are different molecules and the results with one antibody may not parallel results with another. Thus, there is still hope that this mechanism can prove viable for malignant melanoma. Clearly, immunotherapy approaches to cancer are still in their infancy. There are tantalizing results hinting at the promise of such treatments, but a lot more will be learned from ongoing studies to understand if this promise can be fulfilled.

The third area of research, and one that has been exploding with new treatments in the clinic, is an area known as targeted therapies. A great deal is now known about the genetics that drives tumor proliferation. Genes have been identified that drive tumor growth, that suppress tumor growth, or that even induce tumor cell death. These pathways point to new treatments that are specific for tumor cells. The first of these agents have already reached the market such as Genentech's Herceptin® for a specific type of breast cancer, Gleevec from Novartis to treat chronic myeloid leukemia, or Genentech/OSI's Tarceva® to treat non-small-cell lung and pancreatic cancer. But this is simply the beginning. A recent article in *Forbes* magazine showed that the five major pharmaceutical companies in oncology research (Pfizer, Astra-Zeneca, Genentech, Novartis, and GSK) have 72 anticancer agents in clinical development.[15] But, according to PhRMA, when one includes the pipelines of all pharmaceutical companies and biotech companies, there are 750 anticancer compounds in development.

Not all of these compounds will prove to be sufficiently safe and effective for approval. However, with that many in development, more than a hundred are likely to make it. Imagine, a hundred new medicines to treat cancer! This bounty could possibly make cancer a controllable disease. One can envision in the future that a patient diagnosed with a specific cancer will be given the following medications: a targeted anticancer agent specific to the genetic mutation that is causing the tumor's growth; an anti-angiogenesis agent, and an agent to upregulate one's immune system. This isn't science fiction, nor is it going to take 25 years to occur. This scenario could become a reality in the next decade as these hundreds of compounds wend their way through development and approval. And it is important to remember that all of this is rooted in the decades of research funded by the NCI in the War on Cancer.

New cancer drugs will be just one benefit delivered by the pharmaceutical industry in the next 10 years. Hopefully, drugs to treat infectious disease, pain, arthritis, Alzheimer's disease, obesity, diabetes, and other illnesses will also become available. The industry has adjusted to contraction, to increased regulatory oversight, and to commercial hurdles. All of these changes should lead to a renaissance as to how Big Pharma is viewed.

It is not fashionable to view Big Pharma as an industry with a bright future. In fact, skeptics would argue that I am being overly optimistic, and I have certainly been viewed that way in the press.[16] But as a scientist, I am trained to be neither optimistic nor pessimistic. Scientists simply accumulate data and then analyze the results. There is no doubt that the pipelines of most companies are larger than they have ever been. Furthermore, the biotech industry is also seeing a maturity of their pipelines as well. Even assuming traditional attrition rates, these pipelines will provide a number of exciting breakthrough products in the next decade.

But this chapter is not meant to be a defense of the industry's productivity. Rather, it is meant to show that more and better medicines will be available in the near future to patients around the world. Medicines come from this industry and a healthy pharmaceutical industry can only lead to a healthier world.

CHAPTER 12

FINAL REFLECTIONS

PEOPLE OFTEN ask about how pharmaceutical scientists cope with the repeated failures in drug research. After all, more than 90% of the compounds that enter development never become approved medicines. A discovery scientist can spend a 30-year career without discovering a new medicine. What could possibly motivate someone to choose such a career? This perhaps can be explained with an email I received a number of years ago from a Pfizer colleague, David Leventhal. David's father had been battling malignant melanoma and by 2004 had exhausted all the available options to cure his disease. David had heard about our clinical trial with tremelimumab and asked if he could get his father into the clinical program. We were able to do so and some months later David let me know of his father's progress in the most moving email I ever received.

> It is with great joy and excitement that I write to you today.
>
> Tuesday evening, my father received a call from Dr. Toni Ribas of the Anderson Cancer Center at UCLA, informing him that his latest biopsy showed a significant improvement since his latest infusion of tremelimumab. While there is uncertainty about the future, this recent diagnosis is far and away more encouraging than it was four months ago when I first came to see you.
>
> As you recall, my dad's malignant melanoma had moved into Stage Three and was spreading uncontrollably after unsuccessful treatments with traditional chemotherapy and radiation. Through your guidance, and the help of Bill Slichenmeyer and Jesus Gomez-Navarro, we were able to rapidly enroll my dad in the tremelimumab Phase 2 clinical trial. Since his enrollment, my dad has regularly been traveling between Brooklyn, NY and Los Angeles to receive his treatments to be evaluated by Dr. Ribas' team at UCLA.
>
> There is a wonderful story to be told here about what we do at Pfizer, why we do it, and what it means to be a colleague. It would be an honor and a privilege to tell this story to any and all who'll listen.
>
> In my nine years at Pfizer, I have always taken comfort in knowing that I was contributing to something greater than myself. At no other time has this fact been driven home more profoundly and personally.
>
> We like to say here at Pfizer that "the patient is waiting." Little did I know it would be my father.
>
> With Thanksgiving around the corner, there certainly is a lot to be thankful for.

Drug Truths: Dispelling the Myths About Pharma R&D, by John L. LaMattina
Copyright © 2009 John Wiley & Sons, Inc.

I am thankful that my children get to visit their "Grandpa Bobby."

I am thankful that my mom gets to keep the love of her life.

I am thankful that I get to argue with my dad about politics and the NY Mets' starting line-up.

I am thankful for you and your great kindness to me during such a dark time. You told me, "if we can't do for our own people, then who can we do it for?"

I am thankful for Dr. Slichenmeyer, Dr. Gomez-Navarro, and all the great minds who contribute to our collective mission.

Lastly, I am thankful and truly proud that I can be a part of what we do here at Pfizer.

David's father is still alive today. Fortunately, he was one of those patients who responded very well to tremelimumab. David's note eloquently captures all that pharmaceutical workers strive for: We use our talents in the many disciplines needed to invent and bring to patients valued new medicines. We all appreciate how challenging and frustrating this is. Yet, when it all comes together in the discovery of medicines such as Sutent, Selzentry, Lipitor, Celebrex, and so on, it is incredibly fulfilling.

Thanks to the efforts of the pharmaceutical industry, the wonderful result experienced by David Leventhal's father is played out millions of times on a daily basis around the world. Be it life-saving medicines to treat cancer, new drugs to treat painful arthritis that ease the lives of the elderly, or new antibiotics to treat a child's ear infection, this industry is a source of hope. It is time that people recognize the pharmaceutical industry for its contributions and support it in the quest to take health care to a higher level.

REFERENCES

Part I. A Matter of the Heart

1. O'Connor, C. M., Dunne, M. W., Pfeffer, M. A., Muhlestein, J. B., Yao, L., Gupta, S., Benner, R. J., Fisher, M. R., and Cook, T. D. (2003). Azithromycin for the secondary prevention of coronary heart disease events. *Journal of the American Medical Association* **290**, 1459–1466.
2. Grayson, J. T., Kronmal, R. A., Jackson, L. A., Parisi, A. F., Muhlestein, J. B., Cohen, J. D., Rogers, W. J., Crouse, J. R., Borrowdale, S. L. Schron, E., and Knirsch, C. (2005). Azithromycin for the secondary prevention of coronary events. *New England Journal of Medicine* **352**, 1637–1645.
3. Cannon, C. P., Braunwald, E., McCabe, C. H. Grayson, J. T., Muhlestein, B., Giugliano, R. P., Cairns, R., and Skene, A. M. (2005). Antibotic treatment of *Chlamydia pneumoniae* after acute coronary syndrome. *New England Journal of Medicine* **352**, 1646–1654.

Chapter 1. Cholesterol Drugs Are Unnecessary

1. An excellent overview of the early history of this field is: Steinberg, D., and Gotto, A. M. (1999). Preventing coronary artery disease by lowering cholesterol levels; fifty years from bench to bedside. *Journal of the American Medical Association* **282**, 2043–2050.
2. Moore, T. J. (1989). The cholesterol myth. *The Atlantic Monthly* **264**, 37.
3. Castelli, W. P. (1984). Epidemiology of coronary heart disease: The Framingham study. *American Journal of Medicine* **76**(Suppl 2A), 4–12.
4. Lipid Research Clinics Program (1984). The Lipid Research Clinics Coronary Primary Prevention Trial Results. *Journal of the American Medical Association* **251**, 351–374.
5. NIH Consensus Development Conference (1985). Lowering blood cholesterol to prevent heart disease: NIH Consensus Development statement. *Nutritional Reviews* **43**, 283–291.
6. Tolbert, J. A. (2003). Lovastatin and beyond: The history of the HMG-CoA reductase inhibitors. *Nature Reviews, Drug Discovery* **2**, 517–526.
7. These patients are known to have heterozygous familial hypercholesterolemia. This is a relatively common genetic disorder occurring in about 0.2% of the population. These patients have reduced ability for their liver to remove LDL cholesterol from the blood. As a result, they have LDL levels on the order of 300–400 mg/dL and are at the risk of premature heart disease.
8. Brown, M. S., and Goldstein, J. L. (1986). A receptor mediated pathway for cholesterol homeostasis. *Science* **232**, 34–47.
9. Scandinavian Simvastatin Survival Study Group Randomized (1994). Trial of cholesterol lowering in 4444 patients with coronary heart disease: The Scandinavian simvastatin survival study (4S). *The Lancet* **344**, 1383–1389.
10. Oliver, M., Poole-Wilson, P., Shepherd, J., and Tikkanen, M. J. (1995). Lower patients' cholesterol now! *British Medical Journal* **310**, 2180–1281.
11. Zetia® is a registered trademark of MSP Marketing Services © LLD.
12. Vytorin® is a registered trademark of MSP Marketing Services © LLD.
13. IMPROVE-IT, as well as other Vytorin studies, are summarized at www.clinicaltrials.gov.
14. "Merck and Schering-Plough respond to issues raised about ENHANCE clinical trial" Press Release, January 14, 2008.

Drug Truths: Dispelling the Myths About Pharma R&D, by John L. LaMattina
Copyright © 2009 John Wiley & Sons, Inc.

15. Kastelein, J. J. P., Akdim, F., Stoes, E. S. G., Zwinderman, A. H., Bots, M. L., Stalenhoef, A. F. H., Visseren, F. L. J., Sijbrands, E. J. G., Trip, M. D., Stein, E. A., GauDet, D., Duivenvoorden, R., Veltri, E. P., Marais, A. D., and De Groot, E. (2008). Simvastatin with or without ezetimibe in familial hypercholesterolemia. *New England Journal of Medicine* **358**, 1431–1443.
16. Berenson, A. (2008). Cholesterol as a danger has its skeptics. *New York Times*, January 17.
17. Carey, J. (2008). Do cholesterol drugs do any good? *Business Week*, January 28.
18. Greenland, P., and Lloyd-Jones, D. (2008). Critical Lessons from the ENHANCE trial. *Journal of the American Medical Association* **299**, 953–955.
19. These data can be reviewed on the CDC website: www.cdc.gov.

Chapter 2. Industry Is More Interested in "Me-Too" Drugs than in Innovation

1. Lansbury, P. (2003). An innovative drug industry? Well, no. *The Washington Post*, November 16.
2. DiMasi, J. A., and Paquette, C. (2004). The economics of follow-on drug research and development. Trends in entry rates and timing of development. *Pharmacoeconomics* **22**(Suppl 2), 1–14.
3. Goldammer, A., Wiltschnig, S., Heinz, G., Jansen, M., Stulnig, T., Hrl, W. H., and Derfler, K. (2002). Atorvastatin in low-density lioprotein aphaeresis-treated patients with homozygous and heterozygous familial hypecholesterolemia. *Metabolism* **51**, 976–980.
4. LaRosa, J. C., Grundy, S. M., Waters, D. D., Shear, C., Bater, P., Fruchat, J.-C., Gotto, A. M., Green, H., Kastelein, J. J. P., Sheherd, J., and Wenger, N. K., for the Treating to New Targets (TNT) Investigators. (2005). Intensive lipid lowering with atorvastatin in patients with stable coronary disease. *New England Journal of Medicine* **352**(14), 1425–1435.
5. Colhoun, H. M., Betteridge, D. J., Durrington, P. N., Hitman, G. A., Neil, A. W., Livingston, S. J., Thompson, J. J., Mackness, M. I., Charlton-Menys, V., and Fuller, J. H. (2004). Primary prevention of cardiovascular disease with atorvastatin in type 2 diabetes in the Collaborative Atorvastatin Diabetes Study (CARDS): Multicentre randomized placebo-controlled trial. *The Lancet* **364**, 685–696.
6. Sever, P. S., Dahlof, B., Poulter, N. R., Wedel, H., Beevers, G., Caulfield, M., Collins, R., Kjeldsen, S. E., Kristinsson, A., McInnes, G. T., Mehlsen, J., Nieminen, M., O'Brien, E., and Ostergren, J. (2003). Prevention of coronary and stroke events with atorvastatin in hypertensive patients who have average to lower-than-average cholesterol concentrations, in the Anglo-Scandinavian Cardiac Outcomes Trial—Lipid Lowering Arm (ASCOT-LLA): A multicentre randomised controlled trial. *The Lancet* **361**, 1149–1158.
7. Novela, C., and Hennekens, C. H. (2004). Hypothesis: Atorvastatin has pleiotropic effects that translate into early clinical benefits on cardiovascular disease. *Journal of Cardiovascular Pharmacology and Therapeutics* **9**, 61–63.
8. Castro, P. F., Miranda, R., Verdejo, H. E., Greig, D., Gabrielli, L. A., Alcaino, H., Chiong, M., Bustos, C., Garcia, L., Mellado, R., Vukasovic, J. L., Godoy, I., and Lavandero, S. (2008). Pleiotropic effects of atorvastatin in heart failure: Role in oxidative stress, inflammation, endothelial funciton and exercise capacity. *Journal of Heart and Lung Transplantation* **27**, 435–441.
9. Grundy, S. M., Cleeman, J. I., Merz, C. N. B., Brewer, Jr., H. B., Clark, L. T., Hunninghake, D. B., Pasternak, R. C., Smith, Jr., S. C., and Stone, N. J. (2004). Implications of recent clinical trials for the National Cholesterol Education Program Adult Treatment Panel III Guidelines. *Circulation* **110**, 227–239.

Chapter 3. It Takes Industry Too Long to Discover New Drugs

1. American Heart Association, *Heart Disease and Stroke Statistics*, 2005 Update.
2. Franceschini, G. (2000). *American Journal of Cardiology* **88**(Suppl), 9–13.
3. Inazu, A., Brown, M. L., Hesler, C. B., Agellon, L. B., Koizumi, J., Takata, K., Maruhama, Y., Mabuchi, H., and Tall, A. R. (1990). Increased high-density lipoprotein levels caused by a common cholesteryl-ester transfer protein gene mutation. *New England Journal of Medicine* **323**, 1234–1238.

4. (a) Avorn, J. (2005). Torcetrapib and atorvastatin—Should marketing drive the research agenda? *New England Journal of Medicine* **352**, 2573–2576. (b) Shear, C. L. (2005). Torcetrapib and atorvastatin. *New England Journal of Medicine* **353**, 1527.
5. *Pfizer 2001 Annual Report*, page 17.
6. DiMasi, J. A., Hansen, R. W., and Grabowski, H. G. (2003). The price of innovation: New estimates of drug development costs. *Journal of Health Economics* **22**, 151–185.
7. "The Today Show," September 2, 2004.
8. Psaty, B. M., and Lumley, T. (2008). Surrogate end points and FDA approval. A tale of 2 lipid-altering drugs. *Journal of the American Medical Association* **299**, 1474–1476.
9. (a) Kastelein, J. J., Bots, M. L., Visseren, F. L., Evans, G. W., Riley, W. A., Reykin, J. H., Tegeler, C. H., Shear, C. L., Duggan, W. T., Vicari, R. M., and Grobbee, D. E. Torcetrapib and carotid intima-media thickness in mixed dyslipidaemia (RADIANCE 2 study): A randomized, double-blind trial. *The Lancet* **370**, 153–160. (b) Mazzone, T. (2007). *The Lancet* **370**, 107–108. (c) Kastelein, J. J., van Leuven, S. I., Burgess, L., Evans, G. W., Kiuvenhoven, J. A., Barter, P. J., Revkin, J. H., Grobbee, D. E., Riley, W. A., Shear, C. L., Duggan, W. T., and Bots, M. L., for the RADIANCE Investigators (2007). Effect of torcetrapib on carotid atherosclerosis in familial hypercholesterolemia. *New England Journal of Medicine* **356**, 1620–1630.
10. Nissen, S. E., Tardif, J.-C., Nicholls, S. J., Revkin, J. H., Shear, C. L., Duggan, W. T., Ruzyllo, W., Bachinsky, W. B., Lasala, G. P., and Tuzcu, E. M., for the ILLUSTRATE Investigators (2007). Effect of torcetrapib on the progression of coronary atherosclerosis. *New England Journal of Medicine* **356**, 1304–1315.
11. *Medical News Today*, April 3, 2007.

Chapter 4.   Drugs Are Discovered by Academia

1. "The Today Show," September 2, 2004.
2. Consensus Research Stakeholder Value Research, General Public, Phase II, July 2003.
3. Department of Human and Health Services, NIH, Report to Congress on Request to Protect Taxpayers Interests, July 2001.
4. Department of Human and Health Services, NIH, Report to Congress on Affordability of Inventions and Products, July 2004.
5. Morrissey, S. R. Marching in on NIH-funded drugs. *Chemical and Engineering News*, September 14, 2004.
6. Zycher, B., DiMasi, J. A., and Milne, C.-P. (2008). The truth about drug innovation: Thirty-five summary case histories on private sector contributions to pharmaceutical science, Manhattan Institute for Policy Research, Policy Report No. 6, June 2008, www.manhattan-institute.org/html/mpr_06.htm.
7. Kawamura, M., McVicar, D. W., Johnston, J. A., Blake, T. B., Chen, Y., Lal, B. K., Lloyd, A. R., Kelvin, D. J., Staples, J. E., Ortaldo, J. R., and O'Shea, J. J. (1994). Molecular cloning of L-JAK, a Janus family protein-tyrosine kinase expressed in natural killer cells and activated leukocytes. *Proceedings of the National Academy of Science* **91**, 6374–6378.
8. (a) Zhou, Y.-J., Chen, M., Cusack, N. A., Kimmell, L. H., Magnuson, K. S., Boyd, J. G., Lin, W., Roberts, J. L., Lengi, A., Buckley, R. H., Geahlen, R. L., Candott, F., Gadina, M., Changelian, P. S., and O'Shea, J. J. (2001). Unexpected effects of FERM domain mutations on catalytic activity of Jak3: Structural implication for Janus kinases. *Cell* **8**, 959–969. (b) Zhou, Y.-J., Hanson, E. P., Chen, Y.-Q., Magnuson, K., Chen, M., Swann, G., Wange, R. L., O'Shea, J. J., and Changelian, P. S. (1997). Distinct tyrosine phosphorylation sites in JAK3 kinase domain positively and negatively regulate its enzymatic activity. *Proceedings of the National Academy of Science* **94**, 13850–13855.
9. (a) Noguchi, M., Nakamura, Y., Russell, S. M., Ziegler, S. F., Tsang, M., Cao, X., and Leonard, W. J. (1993). Interleukin-2 receptor γ chain: A functional component of the interleukin-7 receptor. *Science* **262**, 1877–1880. (b) Russell, S. M., Keegan, A. D., Harada, N., Nakamura, Y., Noguchi, M., Leland, P., Friedmann, M. C., Miyajima, A., Puri, R. K., Paul, W. E., and Leonard, W. J. (1993). Interleukin-2 receptor γ chain: A functional component of the interleukin-4 receptor. *Science* **262**, 1880–1883.
10. Russell, S. M., Tayebi, N., Nakajima, H., Riedy, M. C., Roberts J. L., Aman, M. J., Migone, T.-S., Noguchi, M., Markert, M. L., Buckley, R. H., O'Shea, J. J., and Leonard, W. J. (1995). Mutation of

JAK3 in a patient with SCID: Essential role of JAK3 in lymphoid development. *Science* **270**, 797–800.

11. Borie, D. C., Changelian, P. S., et al. (2003). Prevention of organ allograft rejection by a specific Janus kinase 3 inhibitor. *Science* **302**, 875–878.

Chapter 5.   New Medicines Add Costs but Little Benefit

1. Soumerai, S. B., McLaughlin, T. J., Ross-Degnan, D., Casteris, C. S., and Bollini, P. (1994). Effects of limiting Medicaid drug-reimbursement benefits on the use of psychotropic agents and acute mental health services by patients with schizophrenia. *New England Journal of Medicine* **331**, 650–655.

2. Cranor, C. W., Bunting, B. A., and Christensen, D. B. (2003). The Asheville Project: Long-term clinical and economic outcomes of a community pharmacy diabetes care system. *Journal of the American Pharmacists Association* **43**(2), 173–184.

3. Bozzette, S. A., Joyce, G., McCaffery, D. F., Leibowitz, A. A., Morton, S. C., Berry, S. H., Rastegar, A., Timberlake, D., Shapiro, M. F., and Goldman, D. P. (2001). Expenditures for the care of HIV-infected patients in the era of highly active antiretroviral therapy. *New England Journal of Medicine* **334**, 817–823.

4. King James I. (1604). *A Counterblaste to Tobacco.*

5. Rollema, H., Chambers, L. K., Coe, J. W., Glowa, J., Hurst, R. S., Lebel, L. A., Lu, Y., Mansbach, R. S., Mather, R. J., Rovetti, C. C., Sands, S. B., Schaeffer, E., Schulz, D. W., Tingley, F. D., III, and Williams, K. E. (2007). Pharmacological profile of the α4β2 nicotinic acetylcholine receptor partial agonist varenicline, an effective smoking cessation aid. *Neuropharmacology* **52**, 985–994.

6. Coe, J. W., Brooks, P. R., Vetelino, M. G., Witz, M. C., Arnold, E. P., Huang, J., Sands, S. B., Davis, T. I., Lebel, L. A., Fox, C. B., Shrikhande, A., Heym, J. H., Schaeffer, E., Rollema, H., Lu, Y., Mansbach, R. S., Chambers, L. K., Rovetti, C. C., Schulz, D. W., Tingley, D., III, and O'Neill, B. T. (2005). Varenicline: An α4β2 nicotinic receptor partial agonist for smoking cessation. *Journal of Medicinal Chemistry* **48**, 3474–3477.

7. *FDA News* (2008). FDA Issues Public Health Advisory on Chantix (February 1, 2008) www.fda.gov/cder/drug/infopage/varenicline/default.htm.

8. Dunlevy, S. (2007). $480 for quit pill. *Daily Telegraph*, November 13.

Chapter 6.   Big Pharma Has Failed and Should Learn From Biotech Success

1. Pisano, G. P. (2006). *Science Business*, Harvard Business School Press, Boston.

2. *National Center for Health Statistics, Centers for Disease Control* Available at http://www.cdc.gov/nchs.

3. Deng, H. K., Liu, R., Ellmeier, W., Choe S., Unutmaz, D., Burkhart, M., DiMarzio, P., Marmon, S., Sutton, R. E., Hill, C. M., Davis, C. G., Peiper, S. C., Schall, T. J., Littman, D. R., and Landau, N. R. (1996). Identification of a major co-receptor for primary isolates of HIV-1. *Nature* **381**, 661–666.

4. Jenkins, R. (2005). How horrors of the plague made Europe safer from AIDS scourge. *The Times (London)*, March 11.

5. Galvani, A. P., and Slatkin, M. (2003). Evaluating plague and smallpox as historical selective pressures for the CCR5-Δ32 HIV-resistance allele. *Proceedings of the National Academy of Sciences* **100**, 15276–15279.

6. Williams, J. A., and Pereira, D. A. (2007). Origin and evolution of high throughput screening. *British Journal of Pharmacology*, 1–9.

7. Dorr, P., Westby, M., Dobbs, S., Griffin, P., Irvine, B., Macartney, M., Mori, J., Rickett, G., Smith-Burchenell, C., Napier, C., Webster, R., Armour, D., Price, D., Stammen, B., Wood, A., and Perros, M. (2005). Maraviroc (UK-427,857), a potent, orally bioavailable and selective small molecule inhibitor of a chemokine receptor CCR5 with broad-spectrum anti-human immunodeficiency virus type 1 activity. *Antimicrobial Agents and Chemotherapy* **49**, 4721–4732.

8. In Europe and other parts of the world, Selzentry is sold as Celsentri.

9. www.Incyte.com/ProductPipeline.

Chapter 7. The Industry Invents Diseases

1. Moynihan, R., Heath, I., and Henry, D. (2002). Selling sickness: The pharmaceutical industry and disease mongering. *British Medical Journal* **324**, 886–891.
2. (a) Petersen, M. (2008). *Our Daily Meds: How the Pharmaceutical Companies Transformed Themselves into Slick Marketing Medicines and Hooked the Nation on Prescription Drugs.* Farrar, Straus and Giroux, New York. (b) Abramson, J. (2004). *Overdosed America: The Broken Promise of American Medicine*, HarperCollins, New York. (c) Cohen, J. S. (2001). *Overdose: The Case Against the Drug Companies*, Penguin, New York.
3. Hulisz, D. (2004). The burden of illness of irritable bowel syndrome: Current challenges and hope for the future. *Journal of Managed Care Pharmacy* **10**, 299–309.
4. Yehuda, R. (2002). Post-traumatic stress disorder. *New England Journal of Medicine* **346**, 108–114.
5. Horowitz, M. (1976). *Stress Response Syndromes*, Aronson, Inc., New York.
6. *Diagnostic Statistical Manual of Mental Disorders, 4th Edition: DSM-IV*, American Psychiatric Association, Washington, DC. 1994.
7. Davidson, J. R. T., Rothbaum, B. O., van derKolk, B. A., Sikes, C. R., and Farfel, G. M. (2001). Multicenter, Double-blind comparison of Sertraline and placebo in the treatment of posttraumatic stress disorder. *Archives of General Psychiatry* **58**, 485–492.
8. Brady, K., Pearlstein T., Asnis, G. M., Baker, D., Rothbaum, B., Sikes, C. R., and Farfel, G. M. (2000). Efficacy and safety of Sertraline treatment of posttraumatic stress disorder. *Journal of the American Medical Association* **283**, 1837–1844.
9. Friedman, M. J., Marmar, C. R., Baker, D. G., Sikes, C. R., and Farfel, G. M. (2007). Randomized double-blind comparison of sertraline and placebo for posttraumatic stress disorder in a Department of Veterans Affairs setting. *Journal of Clinical Psychiatry* **68**, 711–720.
10. Hobson, K. (2007). Gain against the pain. Fibromyalgia knowledge and treatment have improved. *US News and World Report*, October 18.
11. Mease, P. (2005). Fibromyalgia syndrome: Review of clinical presentation, pathogenesis, outcome measures, and treatment. *Journal of Rheumatology* **32**(Suppl 75), 6–21.
12. Crofford, L., Simpson, S., Young, J., Haig, G., and Barrett, J. (2007). Fibromyalgia relapse evaluation and efficacy for durability of meaningful relief (FREEDOM) trial: A six-month, double-blind, placebo-controlled trial of treatment with pregabalin. *Journal of Pain* **8**(Suppl 1), S24.

Chapter 8. New Drugs Are Less Safe Than Traditional Medicines

1. Ricks, D. (2008). List of problem prescription drugs is growing. *Newsday*, January 21.
2. Sharfstein, J. M., North, M., and Serwint, J. R. (2007). Over the counter but no longer under the radar—Pediatric cough and cold medications. *New England Journal of Medicine* **357**, 2321–2324.
3. Lee, W. M. (2004). Acetaminophen and the U.S. Acute Liver Failure Study Group: Lowering the risks of hepatic failure. *Hepatology* **40**, 6–9.
4. Stipp, D. (2006). Take two possibly lethal pills and call me in the morning. *Fortune*, February 20.
5. Three excellent reviews on this topic are: (a) Vane, J. R., Bakhle, Y. S., and Botting, R. M. (1998). Cyclooxygenases 1 and 2. *Annual Reviews of Pharmacology & Toxicology* **38**, 97–120. (b) Maziasz, T., Khan, K. N., Talley, J., Gierse, J., and Seibert, K. (2003). The development of drugs that target cyclooxygenase-2, in *COX-2 Blockade in Cancer Prevention and Therapy*, edited by R. E. Harris, Humana Press, Totowa, NJ, Chapter 16, pp. 259–277. (c) Chandrasekharan, N. V., Dai, H., Roos, L. T., Evanson, N. K., Tomsik, J., Elton, T. S., and Simmons, D. L. (2002). COX-3: A cyclooxygenase variant inhibited by acetaminophen and other analgesic/antipyretic drugs: Cloning, structure and expression. *Proceedings of the National Academy of Sciences* **99**(21), 13926–13931.
6. Gans, K. R., Galbraith, W., Roman, R. J., Haber, S. B., Kerr, J. S., Schmidt, W. K., Smith, C., Hewes, W. E., and Ackerman, N. R. (1990). Antiinflammatory and safety profile of DuP-697, a novel orally

effective prostaglandin synthesis inhibitor. *Journal of Pharmacology and Experimental Therapeutics* **254**, 180–187.

7. Simon, L. S., Weaver, A. L., Graham, D. Y., Kivitz, A. J., Lipsky, P. E., Hubbard, R. C., Isakson, P. C., Verburg, K. M., Yu, S. S., Zhao, W. W., and Geis, G. S. (1999). Antiinflammatory and upper gastrointestinal effects of Celecoxib in rheumatoid arthritis. A randomized controlled trial. *Journal of the American Medical Association* **282**, 1921–1928.

8. Bresalier, R. S., Sandler, R. S., Quan, H., Bolognese, J. A., Oxnius, B., Horgan, K., Lines, C., Riddell, R., Morton, D., Lanas, A., Konstam, M. A., and Baron, J. A., for the APPROVe Trail Investigators (2005). Cardiovascular events associated with Rofecoxib in a colorectal adenoma chemoprevention trial. *New England Journal of Medicine* **352**, 1092–1102.

9. Solomon, S. D., McMurray J. J. V., Pfeffer, M. A., Wittes, J., Fowler, R., Finn, P., Anderson, W. F., Zauber, A., Hawk, E., Bertagnolli, M., for the APC Study Investigators (2005). Cardiovascular risk associated with Celecoxib in a clinical trial for colorectal adenoma prevention. *New England Journal of Medicine* **352**, 1071–1080.

10. ADAPT Research Group (2006). Cardiovascular and cerebrovascular events in the randomized, controlled Alzheimer's Disease Antiinflammatory Prevention Trial (ADAPT). *Public Library of Science Clinical Trials1:e33* (http://dx.doi.org/10.1371/journal.pctr.0010033).

11. For two examples of such studies see: (a) Hippisley-Cox, J., Coupland, C. (2005). Risk of myocardial infarction in patients taking cyclo-oxygenase-2 inhibitors on conventional non-steroidal anti-inflammatory drugs: population based nested case-control analysis. *British Medical Journal* **330**, 1366–1372. (b) McGettigan, P., and Henry, D. (2006). Cardiovascular risk and inhibition of cyclo-oxygenase. A systematic review of the observational studies of selective and nonselective inhibitors of cyclooxygenase 2. *Journal of the American Medical Association* **296**, 1633–1644.

12. www.clinicaltrials.gov Identifier: NCT00346216.

13. Olsen, N. J. (2005). Tailoring arthritis therapy in the wake of the NSAID crisis. *New England Journal of Medicine* **353**, 2578–2580.

Chapter 9.   Industry Spends More on Advertising Than R&D

1. Appleby, J. (2008). As ads surge, more get Rx's filled. *USA Today*, March 4.

2. Congressional Budget Office (2006). Research and Development in the Pharmaceutical Industry Publication No. 2589, Washington, DC, October.

3. Data based on the Pharmaceutical Research and Manufacturers of America Annual Survey of 2006.

4. Koizumi, K. (2007). An Update on the FY 2008 R&D Budget AAAS R&D Budget and Policy Program, http://www.aaas.org/spp/rd.

5. Pharmaceutical Research and Manufacturers of America (2008). *Pharmaceutical Industry Profile 2008*, PhRMA, Washington, DC.

6. (a) Gagnon, M. A., and Lexchin, J. (2008). The cost of pushing pills: A new estimate of pharmaceutical promotion expenditures in the United States. *Public Library of Science Medicine* **5**(1), e1dol:10.1371/journal.pmed.0050001. (b) Donohue, J. M., Cevasco, M., and Rosenthal, M. B. (2007). A decade of direct-to-consumer advertising of prescription drugs. *New England Journal of Medicine* **257**, 673–681.

7. 10th Annual Survey on Consumer Reaction to DTC Advertising of Prescription Medicines, conducted by *Prevention, Men's Health*, and *Women's Health* with assistance from the FDA's Division—Drug Marketing, Advertising and Communication, May 23, 2007, New York.

8. McGlynn, E. A., Asch, M., Adams, J., Keesey, J., Hicks, J., DeCristofaro, A., and Kerr, E. A. (2003). The quality of healthcare delivered to adults in the United States. *New England Journal of Medicine* **348**, 2635–2645.

9. Aikin, K., Swasy, J. L., and Braman, A. C. (2004). Patient and physician attitudes and behaviors associated with DTC promotion of prescription drugs—Summary of FDA Survey Research Results Final Report. US Department of Health and Human Services, Food and Drug Administration, Center for Drug Evaluation and Research, November 19, 2004, Washington, DC.

10. Pharmaceutical Research and Manufacturers of America (2005). *PhRMA Guiding Principles. Direct to Consumer Advertisement About Prescription Medicines*, PhRMA, Washington, DC.

11. McVary, K. T. (2007). Erectile dysfunction. *New England Journal of Medicine* **357**, 2472–2481.

12. Rosen, R. C., Riley, A., Wagner, G., Osterloh, I. H., Kirkpatrick, J., and Mishra, A. (1997). The international index of erectile dysfunction (IIEF): A multidimensional scale for the assessment of erectile dysfunction. *Urology* **49**, 822–830.

13. Galie, N., Ghofrani, H. A. Torbicki, A., Barst, R. J., Rubin, L. J., Badesch, D., Fleming, T., Parpia, T., Burgess, G., Branzi, A., Grimminger, F., Kurzyna, M., and Simonneau, G., for the Sildenafil Use in Pulmonary Arterial Hypertension (SUPER) Study Group (2005). Sildenafil citrate therapy for pulmonary arterial hypertension. *New England Journal of Medicine* **353**, 2148–2157.

Chapter 10. Industry Does Not Care About Diseases of the Developing World

1. Stiglitz, J. E. (2006). Scrooge and intellectual property rights. *British Medical Journal* **333**, 1279–1280.

2. Barton, N., and Wilhelm, I. (2007). Corporate giving rises modestly. *The Chronicle of Philanthropy* **19**, 1–4.

3. Flanagin, A., and Winkler, M. A. (2006). Theme issue on poverty and human development. *Journal of the American Medical Association* **296**, 2970–2971.

4. Friedrich, M. J., (2007). Ending extreme poverty, improving the human condition. *Journal of the American Medical Association* **298**, 1849–1851.

5. Pandey, P., Sehgal, A. R., Riboud, M., Levine, D., and Goyal, M. (2007). Informing resource-poor populations and the delivery of entitled health and social services in rural India. A cluster randomized controlled trial. *Journal of the American Medical Association* **298**, 1867–1875.

6. Gakidou, E., Oza, S., Fuertes, C. V., Li, A. Y., Lee, D. K., Sousa, A., Hogan, M. C., Vander Horn, S., and Ezzati, M. (2007). Improving child survival through environmental and nutritional interventions. The importance of targeting interventions toward the poor. *Journal of the American Medical Association* **298**, 1876–1887.

7. www.gsk.com/malaria

8. www.novartisfoundation.org

9. www.astrazeneca.com.

10. www.sustainability2006.bayer.com.

11. www.merck.com/cr/enabling_access/developing_world

12. www.diflucanpartnership.org.

13. Lopez, A. D., Mathers, C. D., Ezzati, M., Jamison, D. T., and Murray, C. J. L., editors (2006). *Global Burden of Disease and Risk Factors*, Chapter 3, Table 3.6, Harvard University Press, Cambridge, MA. www.dcp2.org/pubs/gbd/3/table/3.6.

14. www.mectizan.com.

15. Bright, G. M., Nagel, A. A., Bordner, J., Desai, K. A., DiBrino, J. N., Nowakowska, J., Vincent, L., Watrous, R. M., Sciavolino, F. C., English, A. R., Retsema, J. A., Anderson, M. R., Brennan, L. A., Borovoy, R. J., Cimochowski, C. R., Faiella, J. A., Girard, A. E., Girard, D., Harbert, C., Manousos, M., and Mason, R. (1988). Synthesis, *in vitro* and *in vivo* activity of novel 9-deoxo-9a-Aza-homoerythromycin A derivatives; A new class of macrolide antibiotics: The azalides. *Journal of Antibiotics* **41**, 1029–1047.

16. Girard, A. E., Girard, D., English, A. R., Gootz, T. D., Cimochowski, C. R., Faiella, J. A., Haskell, S. L., and Retsema, J. A. (1987). Pharmacokinetic and *in vivo* studies with azithromycin (CP-62,993), a new macrolide with an extended half-life and excellent tissue distribution. *Antimicrobial Agents and Chemotherapy* **31**, 1948–1954.

17. Gladue, R. P., Bright, G. M., Isaacson, R. E., and Newborg, M. F. (1989). *In Vitro* and *In Vivo* uptake of Azithromycin (CP-62,993) by phagocytic cells: Possible mechanism of delivery and release at sites of infection. *Antimicrobial Agents and Chemotherapy* **33**, 277–282.

18. Pliva sells the drug under a different trademark, Sunamed, in Central and Eastern Europe.

19. Cook, J. A. (2008). Eliminating blinding trachoma. *New England Journal of Medicine* **353**, 1777–1779.

20. Solomon, A. W., Harding-Esch, E., Alexander, N. D. E., Aguirre, A., HollAnd, M. J., Bailey, R. K., Foster, A., Mabey, D. C. W., Massae, P. A., Courtright, P., and Shao, J. F. (2008). Two doses of azithromycin to eliminate trachoma in a Tanzanian community. *New England Journal of Medicine* **358**, 1870–1871.
21. (a) Lewis, D., Mulenga, M., Mugyenyi, P., Sagara, I., Wasunna, M., Oduro, A., Sie, A., Tiono, A., Sarkar, S., Kityo, C., Djimde, A., Nambozi, M., Juma, R., Germain, M., Ansah, P., Ouedraogo, A., Aman, R., Kokwaro, G., and Dunne, M. (2007). A Phase 2/3, Randomized, Double Blind, Comparative Trial of Azithromycin Plus Chloroquine Versus Mefloquine for the Treatment of Uncomplicated Plasmodium Falciparum Malaria in Africa. Presented at 5th European Congress of Tropical Medicine & International Health, Amsterdam, The Netherlands, May 24–28, 2007. (b) Chandra, R., Lewis, D., Oduro, A., Mulenga, M., Sagara, I., Sie, A., Tiono, A., Dieng, Y., Oguto, B., Sarkar, S., Ansah, P., Nambosi, M., Djimde, A., Zoungrana, A., Ouedraogo, A., Fall, M., Tina Otieno, L., and Dunne, M. (2007). A Phase 3, Randomized, Open-Label, Comparative Trial of Azithromycin Plus Chloroquine Versus Mefloquine for the Treatment of uncomplicated *Plasmodium falciparum* Malaria in Africa. Presented at 56th Annual Meeting of American Society of Tropical Medicine and Hygiene, Philadelphia, November 4–8, 2007.
22. www.ifpma.org/healthpartnerships.

Part IV.   The Future

1. Jordan, G. E. (2008). Where have all the new drugs gone: Industry's medicine cabinet is running empty on compounds. *The Newark Star Ledger*, January 9.

Chapter 11.   Big Pharma's Day Has Passed

1. Kaitlin, K. I., and Manocchia, M. (1997). The new drug approvals of 1993, 1994 and 1995: Trends in drug development. *American Journal of Therapeutics* **4**, 46–54.
2. *Federal Register* (2007). **72**, 58103–58106, October 12.
3. Schmid, E. F., and Smith, D. A. (2005). Is declining innovation in the pharmaceutical industry a myth? *Drug Discovery Today* **10**, 1031–1039.
4. Barer, S. (2007). Celgene: The pharmaceutical Phoenix. *Chemical Heritage Newsmagazine* **24**, 1–2.
5. Richwine, L., and Heavey, S. (2008). FDA official sees some delays over safety. *Reuters*, May 27.
6. Tufts Center for the Study of Drug Development (2006). New drugs entering clinical testing in top 10 firms jumped 52% in 2003–2005. *Tufts CSDD Impact Report* **8**(3), 1–2.
7. www.merck.com/finance/pipeline.swf   and   www.pfizer.com/files/research/pipeline/2008_0228/pipeline_208_0228.pdf.
8. Haran, C., and DeVita, V. (2005). The view from the top. *Cancer World*, Issue 6, 38–43.
9. Folkman, J. (1971). Tumor Angiogenesis: Therapeutic implications. *New England Journal of Medicine* **285**, 1182–1186.
10. Ferrara, N., Hillan, K. J., Gerber, H-P., and Novotny, W. (2004). Discovery and development of bevacizumab, an anti-VEGR antibody for treating cancer. *Nature Reviews Drug Discovery* **3**, 391–400.
11. SUGEN was a biotech company first acquired by Pharmacia, which later merged with Pfizer Inc.
12. Faivre, S., Demetri, G., Sargenti, W., and Raymond, E. (2007). Molecular basis for sunitinib efficacy and future clinical development. *Nature Reviews Drug Discovery* **6**, 734–745.
13. Motzer, R. J., Hutson, T. E., Tomczak, P., Michaelson, M. D., Bukowski, R. M., Rixe, O., Oudard, S., Negrier, S., Szczylik, C., Kim, S. T., Chen, I., Bycott, P. W., Baum, C. M., and Figlin, R. A. (2007). Sunitinib versus interferon alfa in metastatic renal-cell carcinoma. *New England Journal of Medicine* **356**, 115–124.
14. Demetri, G. D., van Oosteroh, A. T., Garrett, C. R., Blackstein, M. E., Shah, M. H., Verweij, J., McArthur, G., Judson, I. R., Heinrich, M. C., Morgan, J. A., Desai, J., Fletcher, C. D., George, S.,

Bello, C. L., Huang, X., Baum, C. M., and Cesali, P. G. (2006). Efficacy and safety of sunitinib in patients with advanced gastrointestinal stromal tumor after failure of imatinib: A randomised controlled trial. *Lancet* **368**, 1329–1338.

15. Herper, M. (2008). Can cancer cure Pfizer? *Forbes*, June 2.
16. Berenson, A. (2006). Dr. Optimistic. A Pfizer scientist sees research dividends ahead. *New York Times*, July 18.

INDEX

Drug Truths: Dispelling the Myths About Pharma R&D, by John L. LaMattina
Copyright © 2009 John Wiley & Sons, Inc.